VOLUME FIVE ■ NUMBER FOUR ■ DECEMBER 2003

CLINICS IN FAMILY PRACTICE

PROFESSIONAL AND PRACTICE MANAGEMENT SKILLS

Guest Editors:
Jean M. Malouin, MD, MPH, and
Randall T. Forsch, MD, MPH

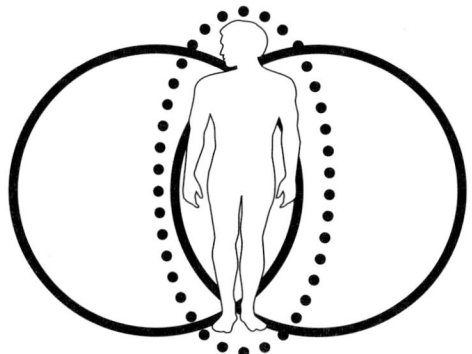

W. B. Saunders Company
A Division of Elsevier Inc.
Philadelphia ■ London ■ Toronto ■ Montreal ■ Sydney ■ Tokyo

W.B. SAUNDERS COMPANY
A Division of Elsevier Inc.

The Curtis Center • Independence Square West • Philadelphia, Pennsylvania 19106
http://www.TheClinics.com

CLINICS IN FAMILY PRACTICE   Volume 5, Number 4
December 2003   ISSN 1522–5720
Editor: J. Heather Cullen

The ideas and opinions expressed in *Clinics in Family Practice* do not necessarily reflect those of the Publisher. The Publisher does not assume any responsibility of any injury and/or damage to persons or property arising out of or related to any use of the material contained in this periodical. The reader is advised to check the appropriate medical literature and the product information currently provided by the manufacturer of each drug to be administered to verify the dosage, the method and duration of administration, or contraindications. It is the responsibility of the treating physician or other health care professional, relying on independent experience and knowledge of the patient, to determine drug dosages and the best treatment for the patient. Mention of any product in this issue should not be construed as endorsement by the contributors, editors, or the Publisher of the product or manufacturers' claims.

Clinics in Family Practice (ISSN 1522–5720) is published quarterly by W.B. Saunders Company. Corporate and Editorial Offices: The Curtis Center, Independence Square West, Philadelphia, PA 19106-3399. **Known Office of Publication**, Accounting and Circulation Offices: 6277 Sea Harbor Drive, Orlando, FL 32887-4800. Subscription prices are $110.00 per year (US individuals), $145.00 per year (US institutions), $55.00 per year (US students), $126.00 per year (Canadian individuals), $175.00 per year (Canadian institutions), $140.00 per year (foreign individuals), $175.00 per year (foreign institutions), and $70.00 per year (foreign students). Foreign air speed delivery is included in all *Clinics* subscription prices. All prices are subject to change without notice. POSTMASTER: Send address changes to *Clinics in Family Practice*, W.B. Saunders Company, Periodicals Fulfillment, Orlando, FL 32887-4800. Customer Service: 1-800-654-2452. (US). From outside of the US, call 1-407-345-4000. E-mail: hhspcs@harcourt.com.

Printed in the United States of America.

CONSULTING EDITOR

BARBARA S. APGAR, MD, MS, Clinical Professor of Family Medicine, University of Michigan Medical School, Chelsea, Michigan

GUEST EDITORS

JEAN M. MALOUIN, MD, MPH, Clinical Assistant Professor, Department of Family Medicine, University of Michigan Medical School, Ann Arbor, Michigan

RANDALL T. FORSCH, MD, MPH, Clinical Assistant Professor, Department of Family Medicine, University of Michigan Medical School, Ann Arbor, Michigan

CONTRIBUTORS

WENDY BIGGS, MD, Clinical Assistant Professor, Department of Family Practice, Michigan State University College of Human Medicine, Lansing; Assistant Director, Midland Family Practice Residency, Midland, Michigan

MARK H. EBELL, MD, MS, Associate Professor, Department of Family Practice, Michigan State University, East Lansing, Michigan

MICHAEL D. FETTERS, MD, MPH, MA, Department of Family Medicine, University of Michigan Health System, Ann Arbor, Michigan

RANDALL T. FORSCH, MD, MPH, Clinical Assistant Professor, Department of Family Medicine, University of Michigan Medical School, Ann Arbor, Michigan

EDWARD B. GOLDMAN, JD, Office of the General Counsel, Health System Legal Office, University of Michigan, Ann Arbor, Michigan

KYLE L. GRAZIER, Professor, Department of Health Management and Policy, School of Public Health, University of Michigan, Ann Arbor, Michigan

FREDERICK W. KRON, MD, Department of Family Medicine, University of Michigan Health System, Ann Arbor; Assistant Director, Family Practice Residency Program, Oakwood Healthcare Systems, Dearborn, Michigan

R. DALE LEFEVER, PhD, Assistant Chair for Planning and Program Development; Assistant Professor, Department of Family Medicine, University of Michigan Health System, Ann Arbor, Michigan

JEAN M. MALOUIN, MD, MPH, Clinical Assistant Professor, Department of Family Medicine, University of Michigan Medical School, Ann Arbor, Michigan

iii

REBECCA A. MALOUIN, PhD, MPH, Epidemiologist, Epidemiology Services Division, Michigan Department of Community Health, Lansing; Fellow, Department of Epidemiology, College of Human Medicine, Michigan State University, East Lansing, Michigan; Instructor, School of Health and Human Services, Walden University, Minneapolis, Minnesota

DEVORAH E. RICH, PhD, Research Investigator, University of Michigan Health System, University of Michigan Medical School, Ann Arbor, Michigan

THOMAS L. SCHWENK, MD, Professor and Chair, Department of Family Medicine; Professor, Department of Medical Education, University of Michigan Medical School, Ann Arbor, Michigan

ERIC SKYE, MD, Clinical Assistant Professor, Department of Family Medicine; Director, Family Practice Residency, University of Michigan Medical School, Ann Arbor, Michigan

QUINTA VREEDE, MHSA, University of Michigan Hospital and Health Centers, Ambulatory Care Services, Ann Arbor, Michigan

REBECCA W. WEST, JD, Executive Director, Piedmont Liability Trust; Assistant Professor of General Medicine, University of Virginia School of Medicine, Charlottesville, Virginia

NEAL WHITMAN, EdD, Professor, Department of Family and Preventive Medicine, University of Utah School of Medicine, Salt Lake City, Utah

LEON WYSZEWIANSKI, PhD, Associate Professor, Department of Health Management and Policy, University of Michigan School of Public Health, Ann Arbor, Michigan

PHILIP ZAZOVE, MD, MM, Clinical Professor, Department of Family Medicine, University of Michigan, Ann Arbor; Associate Medical Director of Ambulatory Care, University of Michigan Hospitals and Health Centers, Dexter, Michigan

Contents

Clinicians, patients, and third-party payers define quality of care in different, but overlapping, terms. This fact explains some of the conflicts and misunderstandings about quality that arise among the three parties and also suggests ways in which the differences can be bridged. Similarly, too many commonly used measures of quality and too many quality-improvement strategies—such as report cards—owe their visibility and currency to the beliefs of one or another influential group rather than to evidence of their validity and utility. Remedying some of the well-documented problems of quality in the United States is most likely to succeed if improvement strategies are chosen based on the best evidence of their efficacy, and if there is explicit recognition that changes must occur at all levels of the system.

This article describes seven skills to help practicing physicians improve their teaching. Family physicians have many opportunities to teach their patients, staff, and colleagues. Some physicians also precept medical students and residents in their offices. All these "learners" in a physician's life will benefit if the physician allows the seven lessons offered in this article to guide his or her educational practice.

This article presents a four-stage model to guide physicians in leadership through the process of managing a change, while keeping the overall organization functioning and maintaining its core values. The four stages to be described include (1) establishing the need, or clarifying the impetus, for the change; (2) understanding and managing resistance to the change; (3) confirming the vision and determining the organization's readiness to make the change; and (4) sustaining the change after initial implementation. Although it is acknowledged that change does not move through these stages at an even or predictable pace, neither can any of these stages or their order be ignored. Planning with these issues in mind, and using these categories to gauge where the organization is in the change process will increase the likelihood of a managed change initiative that achieves its intended purpose.

Family physicians are the first points of contact in the health care system for many individuals and have a great responsibility to identify factors associated with the health status of a patient. Health behavior models provide a framework to identify various components—including demographic, psychosocial, and environmental factors—that may affect a patient's behavior. By selecting an appropriate health behavior model or a combination of models, family physicians can identify specific factors affecting behavior change and the stage of change of a patient, and thus can select an appropriate preventive action or intervention for a patient. Interventions can include individual-level, group-level, community-level, or structural-level components, depending on the needs of a patient and available resources.

Customer satisfaction is paramount to an organization's ability to survive and to thrive in very competitive times. Customers are defined as both internal (employees) and external (patients, employers, referring physicians, and so forth). A strong positive correlation has been noted between employee satisfaction and patient satisfaction. In addition, satisfied staff improve an organization's bottom line by having lower employee turnover. Periodic and consistent measurement of customer satisfaction—through focus groups, one-on-one conversations, or formal surveys that can provide statistically quantifiable feedback—permits organizations to understand the needs of each customer group, and to make process changes that allow organizations to meet and exceed the expectations of their customers.

The Challenging Patient 893
Frederick W. Kron, Michael D. Fetters, and
Edward B. Goldman

On average, about one-sixth of every family physician's patients will challenge their provider's ability to care for them in a productive and satisfying fashion. Often, these are needy individuals in biopsychosocial disequilibrium who lack the insight to understand and communicate their problems in a clear and comprehensible manner. Recognizing these patients when they present, respecting their underlying humanity, and developing communication and coping strategies to deal with them effectively may help to turn an onerous relationship into a rewarding one. Thinking of challenging encounters in a comprehensive way that factors physician self-awareness into the equation also may help to remedy the problem. Finally, in those instances in which the physician-patient relationship is unproductive and cannot be remediated, it may be necessary to terminate it.

Medical-Legal Issues: The Patient Relationship and Risk Management 905
Rebecca W. West

This article discusses the medical—legal issues of the physician–patient relationship, and emphasizes the following seven points: (1) the quality initiative, (2) establishing patient relationships, (3) patient confidentiality and privacy, (4) patient communication, (5) informed consent, (6) medical record practices, and (7) medical malpractice insurance.

Medical-Legal Issues: What You Should Know about the Legal Process 923
Rebecca W. West

This article discusses the medical–legal issues of the legal process, and emphasizes the five following points: (1) the legal process, (2) the standard of care, (3) subpoenas, (4) the stress of litigation, and (5) choosing an attorney.

Health Insurance Systems for Family Physicians 937
Kyle L. Grazier

In the United States, the practice of medicine is linked to the practice of insurance. The language and processes of paying for care permeate the delivery of services. The connection between needing health care and having it available is mediated by a complex system of risk assessment, estimation, and pricing. For family physicians to deliver their services, a basic understanding of who pays and how they pay is essential. This article is a primer on some aspects of a system likely to face physicians and patients in the foreseeable future.

methods to measure and improve efficiency that can be readily used in any clinic.

Physicians, particularly those in primary care, manage large amounts of information every day. As the practice of medicine becomes more complex, challenging, and interrelated, it is more important than ever that physicians develop information management and information technology skills. In this article, we will discuss strategies for keeping up-to-date and answering clinical questions, built around the Information Mastery framework. Key technologies will be reviewed and electronic medical records, decision support systems, and electronic references will be discussed.

Physicians and medical centers around the country face the dual problem of physician access and long wait times. This article discusses clinic scheduling and access techniques that will help physicians to see all the patients who want to be seen on a timely basis, while providing high-quality medical care.

FORTHCOMING ISSUES

RECENT ISSUES

THE CLINICS ARE NOW ONLINE!

Access your subscription at
www.TheClinics.com.

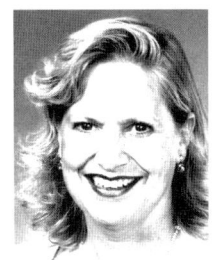
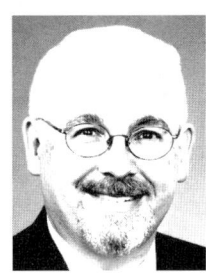

PREFACE

JEAN M. MALOUIN, MD, MPH RANDALL T. FORSCH, MD, MPH
Guest Editors

Many of you may remember the days when being a good physician meant knowing how to take care of patients, period. Success was measured by how good your patients felt and by how much they liked you. What it means to be a physician has changed dramatically over the past few decades, however. The art of medicine is now the science of medicine, and intuition-based medicine has been replaced by evidence-based medicine. Your success is often gauged in terms of Health Plan Employer Data and Information Set (HEDIS) measures and patient satisfaction surveys instead of whether you go home at night feeling like you've brightened a patient's day or improved their health. Not only has the practice of medicine become more complex, being an outstanding clinician alone isn't enough any more—you also have to have business sense.

This concept has been thrust upon all of us in the field of family medicine to some degree. Graduating residents accept it as the norm and comfortably speak the language of relative value units and HEDIS measures as if it were their native tongue. The rest of us are coming around, one way or another, sometimes with enthusiasm and sometimes kicking and screaming. The early adopters are clutching their palm pilots and tablets, quoting Cochrane data at the drop of a hat, and using electronic medical records. The rest of us are clutching our paper charts and trying to figure out how to fit six complex patients into 1 hour. All this while pondering whether our last patient visit "felt" like a level 3 or a level 4 and whether we even have the energy to dictate the supporting documentation for a more complex visit.

Medicine has for generations been referred to as an art; the past two decades have revealed that it is also a business. Traditionally, two camps existed in the delivery of medicine: the physicians who practice it and the administrators who run it. Neither completely understood the other's field of knowledge or the perspective from which it was derived. Physicians would talk of "standard of care" when they needed a new piece of clinical equipment or facility, and administrators would spend the money without completely understanding the medical necessity. The administrators, when they wanted their way, would put up numbers and ratios and the physicians would agree to the plan. The day has come for leaders who possess the knowledge to practice both the art and the business of medicine. These leaders will be physicians who not only provide high quality patient care but also understand the various aspects of finance, management, law, interpersonal skills, and teaching that are necessary to optimize delivery of patient care. These physicians will be able to make complicated decisions by understanding both the medical and the business aspects of the situation. Their eyes will not glaze over when reviewing financial statements, nor will they accept arbitrary quality standards without supportive medical evidence.

Little information now exists as to how physicians learn the business of medicine and develop the expertise necessary to interact with patients, students, and staff within an organizational setting. Residency training hopes to meet this need, frequently using practice management consultants and community-based practice experiences. Much is learned by practical discussion with experienced clinicians who have navigated the billing, financing and office management challenges on their own and have learned "on the fly" or by osmosis. It is our hope that this issue of the *Clinics in Family Practice* will serve as a reference for family medicine residents learning professional and practice management skills as well as practicing physicians who encounter new challenges involving these subjects in their daily experience.

The elements of medicine that are not based on medical knowledge nor taught in medical school are equally important to professional success and satisfaction. The articles in this issue were carefully chosen to fill this knowledge gap. They cover a broad spectrum of topics and can be divided into four main categories: professional skills, physician–patient interactions, financial issues, and office operations.

This issue was created out of a heartfelt understanding and empathy for the complexity surrounding what it means to be a physician today. You are all family physicians because you believe in the concept of comprehensive patient-centered care; at the same time, you are all businessmen and women because you have clinics to run and mortgages to pay. You are educators, negotiators, craftsmen, and scholars. You love what you do and want to be adequately compensated for it.

We are delighted to have been given the opportunity to coedit this issue of the *Clinics in Family Practice* and share some of our experiences. We have been medical directors at our respective clinics for a combined total of 14 years, and 3 years ago received Master of Public Health degrees in health management and policy at the University of Michigan. Somewhere along the line, the business aspects of medicine became our passion, and we are now codirectors of the professional skills component of our residency program at the University of Michigan. This issue represents a departure from the usual medical content found in this publication, and we are grateful for the opportunity to present you with what we hope are some useful tools that you can use throughout your professional career. We are highly indebted to Dr. Barbara Apgar for giving us this opportunity, and to our esteemed colleagues at the University of Michigan and elsewhere, whose contributions have made this issue possible. We are truly fortunate to have been able to work with such outstanding colleagues and to have benefited from their collective experience.

JEAN M. MALOUIN, MD, MPH
RANDALL T. FORSCH, MD, MPH
Guest Editors

Briarwood Family Practice
1801 Briarwood Circle
Ann Arbor, MI 48108
E-mail: jskratek@med.umich.edu

Chelsea Family Practice Center
14700 E. Old US Hwy 12
Chelsea, MI 48118-0738, USA
E-mail: rforsch@med.umich.edu

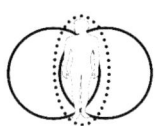

PROFESSIONAL AND PRACTICE MANAGEMENT SKILLS 1522–5720/03 $15.00 + .00

DEFINING, MEASURING, AND IMPROVING QUALITY OF CARE

Leon Wyszewianski, PhD

Quality of care is an increasingly salient issue in dealings between family physicians and third-party payers such as health maintenance organizations (HMOs) and health insurance companies. Third-party payers' notions of what constitutes quality of care can be mystifying and frustrating to the family physician. It turns out, however, that third-party payers also are frustrated by their inability to effectively communicate about quality of care with clinicians, patients, and their employers. It is therefore useful to begin to explore the concept of quality of care by examining how different participants view quality of care, and why they have these views.

WHAT IS QUALITY?

The Clinicians' Definition

The clinicians' view of quality of care is captured in important ways by the often-quoted definition from the Institute of Medicine (IOM) [1]: "Quality is the degree to which health services for individuals and populations increase the likelihood of desired health outcomes and are consistent with current professional knowledge."

Reference to "current professional knowledge" places the assessment of quality of care in the context of the state of the art in clinical care, as opposed to putting it in the realm of more abstract and absolute—and potentially unattainable—expectations. This suits clinicians well; they are much more comfortable with being evaluated in an environment that recognizes that not every ailment can be diagnosed and not every condition can be cured.

From the Department of Health Management and Policy, University of Michigan, School of Public Health, Ann Arbor, Michigan

Similarly, mention of the "likelihood of health outcomes" in the IOM definition implicitly acknowledges the existence of factors that can affect outcomes of care and yet are beyond the clinician's control. The IOM definition also is likely to be congenial to the clinician by its general focus on the technical aspects of care, which include the timeliness and accuracy of diagnosis, the appropriateness of therapy, and the skill with which procedures and other interventions are performed [2,3].

The Patients' Definition

Although patients, like clinicians, are deeply concerned with how good the technical aspect of care is, most do not possess the wherewithal to evaluate the technical elements of care. As a result, patients tend to defer to others on matters of technical quality, and many take for granted that entities that ostensibly possess the requisite expertise and insight— such as licensure and specialty boards—look after technical quality on the public's behalf. As a result, patients tend to form their opinion about quality based on their assessment of those aspects of care that they are more readily able to evaluate: the interpersonal aspect of care and the amenities of care [2,4].

The quality of the interpersonal aspect of care refers to how well the clinician relates to the patient on a human level and, in so doing, fully addresses the patient's concerns. In contrast, the quality of the amenities of care is determined not by what the clinician does, but by the character-istics of the setting in which the interaction between patient and clinician takes place. It relates to such attributes as whether the facilities are appealing and help the patient feel reassured and at ease [2,3]. The notion of amenities also can be extended to include characteristics related to the accessibility of care, such as how readily the clinician can be seen by the patient and how convenient the location of the practitioner's clinic or office is to the patient.

Because patients' reactions to the interpersonal and amenity aspects of care—rather than to the more indiscernible quality of technical aspects—largely determine their level of satisfaction with care, HMOs and other health care organizations have come to view the quality of nontechnical aspects of care as crucial to attracting and retaining patients, often to the dismay of clinicians to whom this is a slight to the centrality of technical quality in the evaluation of medical care.

Another aspect of care that has grown steadily in importance with regard to how patients define quality of care is the extent to which their preferences are taken into account. Although not every patient will have definite preferences in every clinical situation, patients increasingly value being consulted about their preferences, especially in situations in which different approaches to diagnosis and treatment exist that involve potential trade-offs, such as between the quality and the quantity of life. Although clinicians and third-party payers generally express support for respecting and following patients' preferences, in practice they often give primacy to other considerations, such as cost or their own view of potential trade-offs or other concerns and priorities [5].

The Payers' Definition

Third-party payers tend to assess quality of care in the context of costs. From their perspective, quality is unsatisfactory any time the associated costs are higher than they could be. In other words, care that involves waste—in the form of unnecessary use of resources—always is deficient, no matter how good it may be in other respects. Another way in which costs enter into the payers' conception of quality is through the weighing of benefits against costs. Because payers must manage a finite pool of resources on behalf of a group of covered individuals, they have to consider whether a particular potential outcome justifies the associated costs. This is in contrast to the perspective of individual physicians, who generally consider such cost–benefit calculations as antithetic to providing high-quality care. It runs counter to a deep-seated belief that individual physicians are duty bound to do everything possible to help their patients, including advocating for high-cost interventions, even when they have a small, although positive, probability of benefiting the patient [6].

The third-party payer, on the other hand, is more apt to hold the view that spending large sums in instances in which the odds of a positive result are quite small does not represent high quality of care inasmuch as it is a misuse of finite resources. For payers, this has become an especially salient issue as the resources at their disposal become ever more constrained due to the public's growing unwillingness to pay the higher premiums or taxes needed to provide every patient with all the care that is technically feasible and could benefit that individual.

Are the Three Definitions Irreconcilable?

Different though they may seem, the three definitions—the clinicians', the patients', and the payers'—have a great deal in common. Even though each of the definitions clearly emphasizes different aspects of care, it is not to the complete exclusion of the other aspects (Table 1). Only with respect to the cost–benefit aspect can it be said that there is a direct conflict among the definitions. Cost–benefit is central to how payers define quality of care, whereas typically patients and physicians do not recognize it as a legitimate consideration in the definition of quality. However, on all the other aspects of care, no such clash is present; rather, the differences relate to how much weight each definition places on a particular aspect of care.

That is not to say that strong disagreements do not arise among the three parties' definitions, even outside the realm of cost–benefit. Conflicts typically arise when one of the parties holds that a particular practitioner or clinic is a high-quality provider by virtue of having high ratings on a single aspect of care, such as interpersonal quality. Those who object to

TABLE 1.
Importance of Selected Aspects of Care in Key Participants' Definitions of Quality

	Technical	Inter-personal	Amenities	Individual Preferences	Efficiency	Cost–Benefit
Clinicians	+++	+	+	+	+	−
Patients	++	++	++	+++	+	−
Payers	+	+	+	+	+++	++

such a conclusion point out that just because care is high on interpersonal quality does not necessarily mean that it is equally high on the technical, amenity, and efficiency aspects [7]. Physicians who relate especially well to their patients, and thus score high on the interpersonal aspect, still may have failed to keep up with medical advances and, as a result, may provide care that is seriously deficient in technical terms. Conversely, a brilliant diagnostician or a practitioner highly skilled in a particular procedure may have a cold, even brusque, manner that is off-putting to patients, earning that physician low ratings on the interpersonal aspect of care even though the physician gets top marks on technical quality.

In light of these facts, it is important that in order for clinicians, patients, and payers—and any other involved parties—to have a productive dialog about quality of care, they first must recognize explicitly that when they talk about quality of care they each tend to focus on the quality of specific aspects of care, sometimes to the exclusion of other aspects important to the other parties, even though most of the overlooked aspects are not in direct conflict with their own overall concept of quality (see Table 1).

HOW CAN QUALITY BE MEASURED?

Even if clinicians, payers, and patients were to reach a common understanding on how to define quality of care, for such a meeting of minds to be truly meaningful, all three parties would have to agree additionally on how to measure quality. On this score, too, they face hurdles (this issue is discussed later in this article).

Structure, Process, and Outcome

As Donabedian [8] first noted nearly 4 decades ago, all quality of care evaluations can be classified in terms of which of three aspects of caregiving they measure: structure, process, or outcome. When quality is measured in terms of structure, the focus is on the relatively static characteristics of the individuals who provide care and of the settings at which the care is delivered. These include the clinicians' education, training, and board certification; and the facilities' staffing, equipment, and organization.

Evaluations of quality that rely on such structural elements implicitly assume that well-qualified people working in well-appointed and well-organized settings will provide high-quality care. It must be acknowledged, however, that although good structure makes it more likely that good quality will ensue, it does not guarantee it [3]. That is why structure-focused assessments are most revealing when deficiencies are found: good quality is unlikely, if not impossible, if providers are unqualified or necessary equipment is missing or in disrepair. Licensing and accrediting bodies have relied heavily on structural measures of quality because the measures are relatively stable and thus easier to capture, and because they identify reliably those who demonstrably lack the means to provide high-quality care.

Although structural measures of quality make intuitive sense to clinicians, measures that deal with actual caregiving—with the process of care—are even more congenial to clinicians. Process measures capture how appropriate the care was and how skillfully it was provided. Use of process measures in the assessment of quality rests on the expectation that, as it is sometimes put, if the clinician does the right things and does them right, good results will ensue. Those results, in turn, are the focus of outcome measures of quality that seek to capture whether, for example, the pain subsided, the condition cleared up, or full functioning was regained by the patient [2,3].

Clinicians tend to be somewhat leery of outcome measures of quality. They are quite aware that many factors that determine clinical outcomes are not under the clinician's control [9]. They recognize that—as the IOM definition of quality clearly reflects—good process increases the likelihood of good outcomes, but does not guarantee them. Some patients do not get better in spite of the best that medicine can offer, whereas other patients regain full health even though they received inappropriate and potentially harmful care. On the other hand, the relation between process and outcomes is not random or wholly unpredictable—in particular, the likelihood that a specific set of clinical activities, a given process, will result in desirable outcomes depends crucially on how efficacious that process has been shown to be.

Efficacy

A clinical intervention is said to be efficacious if it has been shown to produce reliably a given outcome when other, potentially confounding, factors are held constant [10]. The efficacy of a clinical intervention is established typically through formal clinical trials or similarly systematic and controlled studies. Knowing that a given intervention has been found to be efficacious under a particular set of clinical circumstances makes it possible to answer a question that is critical to the assessment of care: in this specific case, was the right thing done? At least at first approximation, the right thing to do—the care appropriate to the situation—is that which has been shown to be efficacious.

As it turns out, however, determining the appropriateness of care is, in many instances, difficult, because all the requisite information about efficacy is lacking. Although estimates vary, for at least half of what physicians do in their daily practice, efficacy has not been established definitely [11,12]. There is much care provided, therefore, about which it is not possible to make definitive, efficacy-based assessments of quality. Even so, there is reason to believe that, overall, quality of care is not as good as it could be or is believed to be. Within the set of clinical activities for which definitive information on efficacy is available—and for which appropriateness therefore can be measured—the findings are not encouraging [13–15].

What Studies Show About Quality

In 2001, the IOM [14] issued a report proclaiming that a "chasm" exists in US medical care between what we know about appropriateness and safety and what actually is done in practice. The IOM report, entitled *Crossing the Quality Chasm*, called for changes—such as wider adoption of evidence-based practices—aimed at closing the gap between current medical practice and what is known to be efficacious. The IOM report's conclusions and its recommendations are not easily dismissed. They are based on well-designed and well-executed quality-assessment studies of practices for which the evidence about efficacy is most robust, such as the prescribing of beta blockers for patients with heart disease. Moreover, the IOM report is not the first to draw attention to the gap between what is known in medicine and what is actually done in practice. For some time now, analogous facts and findings have been cited in repeated calls for changes in clinical practice and, more recently, for the widespread adoption of evidence-based practices [16–18].

Perhaps the IOM report's most novel aspect is its insistence that, to effectively close the gap between evidence and practice, more needs to be done than to once again exhort physicians to try harder and do better. The IOM report makes clear that many others must do their part for success to be achieved. Third-party payers in particular are urged to do away with payment policies that thwart clinicians' adoption of evidence-based practices to such a degree that they have been described as "toxic payment policies" [19].

In direct response to the IOM's *Quality Chasm* report [14], in early 2003 a group of third-party payers, large employers, and others established the "Bridges to Excellence" program [20], which features several "pay-for-performance" experiments. One of these experiments pays individual physicians a bonus for each patient with diabetes whose care meets specific standards [20]. The standards, in turn, were put together by the

National Committee on Quality Assurance (NCQA), an organization best known for the ubiquitous Health Plan Employer Data and Information Set (HEDIS) measure of quality (described below).

WHAT MEASURES OF QUALITY ARE BEING USED?

When HMOs and other third-party payers talk to clinicians about quality of care, it is often in the context of HEDIS. A major reason that HMOs and other payers are concerned with measuring and reporting on quality of care is to communicate with, and be responsive to, their enrollees' employers—which also is why many plans additionally use the Consumer Assessment of Health Plans (CAHPS), which NCQA requires for its accreditation program of health plans.

The 2003 version of HEDIS consists of 42 individual measures [21]. (Strictly speaking, only the version of HEDIS for "commercial plans" has 42 measures; two other versions of HEDIS, one geared toward Medicaid patients, the other toward Medicare patients, each involve somewhat different numbers, and arrays, of measures.) The 42 measures can be categorized roughly as follows:

- Thirteen are measures of use, mostly of inpatient care services, expressed as numbers of discharges and average lengths of stay for diagnostic categories such as chemical dependency, mental health, births, and delivery. Although this is the single largest group of measures within HEDIS, NCQA's 2002 report on the "State of Health Care Quality" [22] makes no reference to any of them, possibly reflecting the ambiguous relation between most use measures and quality of care. For example, in the absence of other information, it is not clear what longer or shorter lengths of stay say about quality of care; arguably they speak more to concerns about costs of care than about quality.
- Ten are prevention and screening measures, such as the percentage of women in specified age groups screened for breast cancer, cervical cancer, and chlamydia; the percentage of children with up-to-date immunizations; and the percentage of children ages 3 to 6 who had annual well-child visits. In contrast to the measures of use in HEDIS, the relationship to quality of care of this second group is much more straightforward. Their probability of leading to desirable outcomes—their efficacy—is well established as being positive. Additionally, with the possible exception of breast cancer screening, their cost–benefit ratios are not controversial.
- Seven measures focus on the medical management of selected conditions, most of them chronic. These measures tend to be very specific, for example, percentage of post–heart attack patients on beta blockers. A few, however, are more complex, encompassing several submeasures. The most complex is "comprehensive diabetes care," composed of six different percentages, such as

percentage of patients with diabetes who had an HbA1c test in the past year and percentage of patients with low-density lipoprotein cholesterol level controlled to less than 130 mg/dL. The seven medical management measures are highlighted in NCQA's 2002 "State of Health Care Quality" report [22], under the rubric of "effectiveness measures of care," an appropriate designation given that they represent measures whose efficacy, and hence relation to desired outcomes, is well established (eg, beta-blocker treatment after heart attack). Similarly, the outcome measures included in this set—such as control of high blood pressure or cholesterol—are the kinds that reflect reasonably well how appropriate and skillful the antecedent process of care was.

The remaining measures included in HEDIS are either structural measures of quality, such as percentage of physicians who are board certified; relate to accessibility of care; or are descriptive of the plan, such as numbers of persons enrolled for each type of insurance the plan sells. As with use measures, none of these remaining measures are highlighted in NCQA's 2002 report on quality [22], presumably much for the same reason—that is, the extent to which these measures reflect quality of care is open to debate.

CAHPS

The CAHPS originally was developed under federal government auspices and consists of a series of questions designed to determine the level of patients' satisfaction with their health plans' quality of care and level of service. Currently, CAHPS questions focus on ambulatory care; the federal government is spearheading the development of a version of CAHPS specifically aimed at assessing patient satisfaction with inpatient hospital care.

In its 2002 report on quality [22], the NCQA provides results for four CAHPS questions that relate to patients' overall ratings of, respectively, their personal doctor, their specialists, their health care, and the health plan. Although what these ratings actually reflect is apt to vary across individuals—and within individuals, across the four items—both theory and empiric findings suggest that all four ratings are most likely to be based on patients' assessments of the interpersonal aspects of care and amenities of care, and much less on the technical aspects [2,4]. That may explain why most clinicians do not see such ratings as very meaningful indicators of quality, and hence do not share health plans' concerns with raising those ratings to attract new members and retain current ones.

Responses to all other CAHPS questions are grouped in the NCQA's 2002 report on quality [22] into six sets of "composites" of ratings that NCQA labels "getting needed care," "getting care quickly," "how well doctors communicate," "courteousness of office staff," "customer service," and "claims processing." Because these composite measures, and the questions behind them, relate primarily to the quality of access to care, administrative issues, and interpersonal aspects of care rather than to the quality of technical care, they too are unlikely to be seen by clinicians as truly valid indicators of quality of care.

Report Cards

The notion of quality of care "report cards" gained currency in the early 1990s, as part of a renewed desire—reflected in "managed competition" proposals—to rely on competition in the marketplace to improve quality of care while at the same time foster efficiency in the delivery of care [23,24]. This general perspective also was behind the "managed care revolution" that took the health care field by storm during the same time period. The general premise of managed competition (and of "value purchasing," a related concept) is that if individuals and their employers are given ready access to report cards on the quality of care provided by HMOs—or hospitals, individual physicians, or any other providers of care—they will be in a position to choose, and thereby reward with their business, the providers who offer the best value, defined as the highest level of quality for the money [25].

Data from HEDIS and CAHPS figure prominently in the typical HMO report card. Hospital report cards, on the other hand, typically focus on mortality rates, featuring comparisons between observed mortality rates and "expected" rates calculated for the specific hospital, taking into account its case mix. A number of methodologies for calculating expected rates have been developed over the years. These methodologies are, for the most part, proprietary, which has made assessing the meaningfulness of the measures more difficult. Nevertheless, many different studies over the years have raised questions about the validity of such mortality rate reports as indicators of quality [26–28].

Overall, report cards have not as yet fulfilled the hopes and expectations that attended their introduction. A 2001 review [29] of 32 empirical studies of report cards concluded that, "The evidence indicates that consumer report cards do not make a difference in [consumers'] decision-making, improvement in quality, or competition." Many of the reasons for that can be gleaned from the introductory passage to a *Consumer Reports* article [30] on quality of health care:

> If you're looking for an HMO this fall, you can probably find the cheapest plan, but you can't find the best—one whose doctors always make timely and correct diagnoses, choose effective treatments, and avoid mistakes. That's because there are no good comparisons of health plans on measures like these. However, you may be able to find an HMO that answers your phone calls quickly, has reasonably short waits in doctors' offices, offers a large number of board-certified physicians, and gives you a wide choice of practitioners—indicators that the public has come to equate with good medicine in managed care. Often touted in "report cards," those dimensions, while desirable, have little to do with true quality.

Physician Profiles

Although sometimes lumped in with report cards, physician profiles differ from report cards in a number of ways. Whereas the information contained in the typical report card relates to large entities such as an HMO or a hospital, the physician profile is characterized by its focus on individual physicians. Also unlike other report cards, which are intended primarily for public consumption, physician profiles tend to be used internally by health care delivery organizations such as HMOs and hospitals, typically to ensure that individual physicians are providing care at the desired level of quality and efficiency.

Physician profiles also figure prominently in many HMOs' decisions as to which physicians the HMO will continue to contract with. Because of that, physician profiles often reflect the third-parties' definition of quality of care, with an attendant emphasis on aspects of care that ultimately affect costs. This bias is reinforced by the relative paucity of clinical information readily available to those who produce the profiles, and hence their heavy reliance on administrative data, such as number of inpatient admissions and length of stay, numbers of visits, and cost of laboratory tests and medications ordered. Additionally, because normative standards often are unavailable for those kinds of data, the tendency in physician profiles is to compare the profiled physician's data with group averages rather than evidence-based standards. Most of the time the comparisons are made within specific diagnostic categories and are adjusted for age and sex, but sophisticated case-mix adjustments are not the norm.

Because physician profiles often reflect third-party payers' definition of quality, and feature cost and use data drawn from administrative sources, they have few supporters among clinicians, whose definition of quality would dictate that profiles be based on clinical data properly adjusted for case mix, with comparisons to normative, evidence-based standards [31]. In an empiric evaluation of physician profiles, Hofer et al [32] showed that measures typically included in physician profiles for diabetes care were not able to detect reliably true practice differences that affect quality of care. Moreover, they showed that physicians can readily improve the numbers in their profile through tactics that actually could lower the quality of care received by patients, such as avoiding or dropping from their panel patients with high prior cost, poor adherence, or poor response to treatments [32].

The Prospects for Better Measures

From the prototypic clinician's perspective, the kind of widely used measures of quality just discussed—HEDIS, CAHPS, report cards, and physician profiles—leave much to be desired. The measures are driven mostly by third-party payers' definitions of quality that emphasize costs, interpersonal aspects, and amenities, as opposed to the clinicians' overriding concern with technical quality. The measures also suffer from methodologic shortcomings, such as inadequate case-mix adjustments and low reliability.

Unfortunately, many of the measures' shortcomings can be traced to the basic inadequacy of current approaches for recording and storing clinical information. A key reason that only relatively crude case-mix adjustments prevail and that unsatisfactory proxy measures of quality are used is the relative inaccessibility of the detailed clinical information needed to do better. Patient charts—the primary source of clinical information—are still largely mired in nineteenth century pen-and-paper technology, and the experience of the last decade with medical informatics suggests that bringing the medical chart into the twenty-first century is still some time away, given the effort and expense that this will require [14,33].

Nevertheless, for at least some areas of practice there is, as noted earlier, sufficiently reliable and valid quality of care information to fully justify concerted efforts to remedy the deficiencies that have been identified [14,15]. But how should this be accomplished? Not surprisingly, the answer to that question varies depending on who is asked. Clinicians, payers, and policy makers, among others, each have their own perspective on how quality of care should be improved.

WHICH QUALITY IMPROVEMENT STRATEGIES SHOULD BE USED?

The Clinicians' Perspective

Clinicians' first instinct when faced with deficiencies in quality of care is to assume the problem is inadequate knowledge, which can be corrected through education. In general, clinicians prefer to rely on educational interventions to ensure high-quality care. The interventions they favor are epitomized by continuing medical education (CME), but include other modalities, such as grand rounds; dissemination of clinical guidelines; and, most visibly, the publication of medical journals.

The belief in educational interventions has persisted in spite of overwhelming evidence, dating back at least 2 decades, that educational interventions do not produce lasting changes in physicians' clinical practices [34]. Traditional CME, in particular, consistently has been found, in dozens of randomized controlled trials, to not be effective in bringing about lasting changes in clinical behaviors [35–38]. Implementation of practice guidelines has had a similarly unhappy history of failing to change physician behaviors [39].

A variation on education that clinicians find acceptable for remedying quality of care deficiencies, and that administrators often favor, is physicians providing feedback to other physicians about their performance. This method has been found to work reasonably well, but only if the feedback is provided one on one and face to face—as opposed to simply sending physicians written reports about their performance—and only, in many cases, if a respected colleague (an "influential physician") provides the feedback and does so at regular intervals [34,40,41]. Often, however, this is not easy to implement: influential physicians usually are not eager to commit to an indefinite series of meetings with colleagues whose performance is sub par. In addition, paying for the time that these influential physicians devote to providing feedback also can become quite expensive, even prohibitive.

The Payers' Perspective

Given how they approach quality, payers are especially concerned about instances of overuse, characterized by the provision of unnecessary care. Because care that is unnecessary is wasteful and harmful—it subjects the patient to the risks inherent in any medical intervention without any offsetting benefits—in overuse payers' concerns about cost happily intersect with broader concerns about quality. Payers focus less on two other quality problems that have a more ambiguous relation to costs (and, additionally, can be harder to detect with readily available administrative data): underuse, the failure to provide needed care, and misuse, appropriate care provided incorrectly, as when surgical mishaps occur or abnormal laboratory results are not followed up.

To address overuse, payers tend to rely on the incentives (and attendant penalties) inherent in how providers are paid. However, it is a big challenge to devise payment mechanisms that yield the desired results without unintended consequences, a point dramatized by one reviewer of the literature on this topic [42] when he stated that "there are many mechanisms for paying physicians; some are good and some are bad. The three worst are fee-for-service, capitation, and salary." That may explain why payers additionally have relied on a number of administrative mechanisms to control overuse. These mechanisms generally fit under the rubric of "use management." Among them, payers have relied most heavily on utilization review (UR).

UR originally was associated with payers' efforts to control the costs of inpatient hospital use by eliminating unnecessary admissions and shortening lengths of stay. UR typically is obligatory; physicians must submit to case-by-case reviews before admitting a patient to the hospital, and subsequently must get approval for the patient's continued stay. UR later was extended to other areas that payers identified as costly and subject to inappropriate or inefficient use, including referrals to specialists and certain diagnostic and treatment interventions, such as MRIs. Typically, payers contract with an outside UR organization to perform UR.

Although it is estimated that well over half the patients seen by physicians in the United States are subject to some form of UR, and UR has been in wide use for over 2 decades, the evidence on the effects of UR on quality is limited [43]. It is not known to what extent UR actually improves the appropriateness of care, and in fact there is some evidence that UR may have deleterious effects on quality: one set of studies [44–46] involving different patient groups consistently showed that cases in which the UR process resulted in a reduction in the length of stay requested by physicians were significantly more likely to have an increased relative risk of re-admission.

UR and other utilization-management strategies also have been criticized for being too often driven by statistical averages rather than normative, evidence-based clinical standards. This, and the second-guessing and administrative burden inherent in UR, have been the source of profound dissatisfaction among physicians. In large part because of that, UR has fallen into disfavor among HMOs and other payers, as reflected in United Health Care's much-publicized decision in 1999 to replace UR with approaches that seek to increase patients' involvement in their own care and to achieve better coordination of care for chronic diseases and thereby improve both quality and efficiency of care simultaneously. Other payers have followed the lead of United Health Care and adopted, to varying degrees, new forms of utilization management, notably demand management and disease management.

Demand management generally seeks to reduce patients' demand for care by giving them information about what they themselves can do to improve their well-being and by telling them about alternatives to expensive care modalities, particularly when the added cost of a particular modality is not likely to be related to a more desirable process or to better outcomes. Whereas demand management tends to be offered widely to all members of a plan, disease management is targeted very specifically to patients who suffer from, or are at high risk for, chronic conditions, particularly conditions such as arthritis and asthma for which lifestyle and self-care can play a major role, and those, like diabetes, that are likely to require the involvement of several different clinical disciplines. In theory, disease management produces better clinical and quality-of-life results for the patient and lower costs for the payer by encouraging appropriate lifestyle changes and improving the timing and coordination of clinical interventions. However, neither demand management nor disease management have been in use long enough or sufficiently well studied to know if they work as hoped.

The Policy Makers' Perspective

Which quality improvement strategies ultimately are adopted is influenced greatly by a varied group of "policy makers," individuals and groups from within both the private and the public sectors—such as legislators, government officials, organized professional groups, and business coalitions—who often affect the choice of strategies. Among these policy makers, fundamental disagreements often occur between those who favor market-based approaches and those who are inclined toward regulatory remedies.

Advocates of market-based, competitive approaches subscribe to the notion that competitive markets for goods and services reward the most efficient producers, resulting in prices of goods and services that are very close to the minimum cost of production. These market advocates ascribe problems of low quality and high costs in health care to insufficiently competitive markets. To make the market for health care services more competitive—and thereby raise quality and reduce costs—they favor giving individuals (and their employers) the necessary information and incentives to promote shopping for best values in health care. They therefore strongly support the dissemination of report card information as a way of making individuals more savvy shoppers of health care services. They similarly favor restrictions on health insurance—such as substantial deductibles and co-payments—to give individuals an incentive to take costs into account when making decisions about health care, particularly for discretionary services and services that have low cost–benefit ratios.

Advocates of regulatory approaches, on the other hand, argue that expecting consumers to comparison shop for health care is inherently problematic, given the difficulties most people have in assessing the technologic aspects of care that are so central to overall quality. Furthermore, one argument goes, even if meaningful ratings of quality were available and used widely by consumers, waiting for the market to identify and ultimately weed out poor performers implies a willingness to countenance an unpredictably long string of dangerous or even fatal caregiving episodes. That may be why our society does not rely on market forces to eliminate unsafe and dangerous practices in other areas, such as air travel and restaurants; in those areas, governmental regulatory powers are used to ensure—through inspections and the imposition of explicit standards—that planes are safe to fly and restaurant food is safe to eat. So too, the argument goes, should be the case with health care: rather than rely on the workings of the market to ensure that the care provided is of high quality, vigorous use should be made of governmental regulatory powers to prevent harm before it can happen.

Thus, as with definitions of quality, different participants—such as clinicians, payers, and policy makers—have different perspectives on which quality-improvement strategies should be used. That raises the question of how to reconcile them or choose among them.

WHICH PATH TO QUALITY IMPROVEMENT AND CONTROL?

Significantly, the recommendations of the IOM *Quality Chasm* report [14] that deal with how to improve quality of care do not side with any one specific perspective on improvement strategies, including the ones just described. Instead, the recommendations stress that, given the complexity and interrelatedness of our system of health care, action must be taken at all levels of the system to achieve success [14]. In this context, "success" is measured, as one of the report's framers put it [19], "in the experience of patients, their loved ones, and the communities in which they live," which means that improvement actions must encompass all levels of the system that affect the experience of patients. Hence:

- The functioning of the small units of care delivery or "micro-systems," such as a cardiac surgical team or a small clinical office practice, must be altered fundamentally. This is where "the 'quality' experienced by the patient is made or lost" [19]. The *Quality Chasm* report [14] advocates redesigning microsystems to promote prac-tices that are evidence based and "patient centered," in the sense of "providing care that is respectful of and responsive to individ-ual patient preferences, needs and values and ensuring that patient values guide all clinical decisions." This in turn requires major changes in such areas as how clinical information is collected and used, how caregivers relate to one another and to patients, and the role of organizational mechanisms in caregiving.
- However, such restructuring of microsystems can occur only if the organizations that house the microsystems themselves change in ways that promote and support the restructuring of microsystems. This means that the organizations have to evolve and change in areas such as information technology, human resource develop-ment, building of effective teams, and performance assessment.
- Similarly, for the changes to occur at the organizational level, the payment, regulatory, and other policies that shape health care organizations' incentives, rewards, and opportunities also must change, in some cases dramatically. This includes the elimination of the "toxic payment systems" mentioned earlier that undermine the provision of high-quality care [19]. Equally in need of overhaul are any policies—in areas such as capital financing of health care or-ganizations, accreditation, regulation, and professional education—that fail to promote and support the provision of high-quality care.

Additionally, if a key goal of all these changes is to better align physicians' clinical behaviors with evidence-based practices, it behooves the efforts themselves to be evidence driven. However, as Grol and colleagues [47,48] have argued, currently there is too little information about what is and is not efficacious in changing physicians' clinical behaviors. Still, as was already noted, the information that is available, especially with respect to the very limited efficacy of CME and related educational interventions such as the dissemination of guidelines, too often is overlooked. The same evidence also strongly suggests that lasting changes are more likely to occur if barriers to change in specific situations are identified and effectively addressed, and if, in general, one-size-fits-all approaches to improvement are avoided [37,47,49].

At a broad policy level, the cause of improving quality of care also may benefit if the arguments of advocates of market-based approaches and those of proponents of regulation are considered on their merits in specific contexts rather than subscribed to on purely ideologic grounds, such as a blanket belief in market competition and a distrust of government regulation, or the opposite set of beliefs. It may well be that in health, as in other areas, competition and regulation are complements, and each works best in situations in which the other is relatively ineffective. For example, safety issues in commercial aviation are strictly regulated; airlines do not compete on the issue of which has had the fewest number of crashes or near misses in mid-air. At the same time, however, airlines are free to compete on routes, cabin comfort, staff friendliness, and other nonsafety aspects of their services. In health care as well, regulatory approaches may be the best approach for ensuring the quality of technical care, because the stakes are particularly high in the technical area and this is where most consumers are least able to make assessments. In contrast, the interpersonal and amenity aspects of care may improve most effectively if left to market competition, because this is an area that consumers can assess readily based on their own individual preferences.

SUMMARY

The allure of simplicity was no doubt an important factor in humanity's longstanding, but vain, quest for a single etiologic theory of disease, and the parallel search for a panacea. In the quality of care area, there has been a similarly enduring yearning for a single definition of quality and for a universal strategy for remedying deficiencies in quality of care. As in medicine, however, progress in the quality arena depends, in large part, on coming to terms with the complexity inherent in the area. What this means, to start with, is accepting that there is not one definition of quality of care, but several that overlap and even conflict with one another: the clinicians' definition, which centers on technical quality; the patients' definition, which is driven largely by the quality of interpersonal interactions and the amenities of care; and the third-party payers' definition, which gives primacy to efficiency and cost–benefit considerations.

Similarly, with respect to how quality is measured and how quality improvement strategies are adopted, everyone stands to benefit if a clear separation is made between what is backed by sound empiric evidence and what is driven by the preferences, beliefs, and interests of participants such as clinicians, patients, payers, and policy makers, or is the result of a lack of sufficient resources or the relative backwardness of clinical information systems. This separation would make it possible to move away from debating in the abstract the merits of report cards, educational strategies, or regulatory mechanisms and instead focus energy on using what has been learned from the evidence, and work at all levels of the complex health care delivery system that need to change for quality to improve substantially, as the IOM's *Quality Chasm* report [14] so forcefully argues.

Key Points

- Quality of care is not defined in the same way by everyone, because not all aspects are equally important to all. The clinician gives greatest weight to technical quality; the patient, to quality of interpersonal interactions and the amenities of care; and the third-party payer, to efficiency and cost–benefit considerations.
- The most visible measures of quality, such as report cards, tend to reflect a specific view of quality, often the payer's. Regardless of what view of quality is taken, however, development of valid and useful measures of quality is hampered by limited evidence on efficacy of health care interventions and the relative backwardness of clinical information systems.
- Quality of care in the United States is characterized by a substantial gap between what is known about appropriateness and safety and what actually is done in practice.
- For quality of care in the United States to improve, it will not be enough to educate physicians about the latest scientific evidence or to exhort them to try harder. Change also must take place in the many aspects of the overall system that affect quality, such as how care is paid for, how clinical information is collected and used, and how caregiving is organized.

References

[1] Institute of Medicine. Medicare: a strategy for quality assurance. Washington (DC): National Academy Press; 1990.

[2] Donabedian A. Explorations in quality assessment and monitoring. Vol. I: the definition of quality and approaches to its assessment. Ann Arbor (MI): Health Administration Press; 1980.

[3] Donabedian A. The quality of care: how can it be assessed? JAMA 1988;260(12):1743–8.

[4] Cleary PD, McNeil BJ. Patient satisfaction as an indicator of quality care. Inquiry 1988;25(1):25–36.

[5] The SUPPORT Principal Investigators for the SUPPORT Project. A controlled trial to improve care for seriously ill hospitalized patients: the Study to Understand Prognoses and Preferences for Outcomes and Risks of Treatments (SUPPORT). JAMA 1995;274: 1591–8.

[6] Donabedian A. Quality and cost: choices and responsibilities. Inquiry 1988;25(1):90–9.

[7] Wyszewianski L. Quality of care: past achievements and future challenges. Inquiry 1988;25(1):13–22.

[8] Donabedian A. Evaluating the quality of medical care. Milbank Q 1966;(44):166–203.

[9] Iezzoni LI. Risk adjustment for measuring healthcare outcomes. 3rd edition. Chicago: Health Administration Press; 2003.

[10] Williamson JW, Hudson JI, Nevins MM. Principles of quality assurance and cost containment in healthcare. San Francisco (CA): Jossey-Bass; 1982.

[11] Bunker JP. Is efficacy the gold standard for quality assessment? Inquiry 1988;25(1):51–8.

[12] Eddy DM. Three battles to watch in the 1990s. JAMA 1993;270:520–6.

[13] Schuster MA, McGlynn EA, Brook RH. How good is the quality of health care in the United States? Milbank Q 1998;76:517–63.

[14] Institute of Medicine. Crossing the quality chasm: a new health system for the 21st century. Washington (DC): National Academy Press; 2001.

[15] McGlynn EA, Asch SM, Adams T, Keesey T, Hicks T, DeCristofaro A, et al. The quality of health care delivered to adults in the United States. N Engl J Med 2003;348:2635–45.

[16] Cochrane AL. Effectiveness and efficiency: random reflections on health services. London: Nuffield Provincial Hospitals Trust; 1972.

[17] Eddy DM. Clinical decision making: from theory to practice. Sudbury (MA): Jones and Bartlett; 1996.

[18] Evidence-Based Medicine Working Group. Evidence-based medicine. A new approach to teaching the practice of medicine. JAMA 1992;268:2420–5.

[19] Berwick DM. A user's manual for the IOM's "quality chasm" report. Health Aff (Milwood) 2002;21(3):80–90.

[20] Bridges to excellence. Available at: http://www.bridgestoexcellence.org/bte/. Accessed June 7, 2003.

[21] National Committee for Quality Assurance. HEDIS 2003 summary table of measures and product lines. Washington (DC): National Committee for Quality Assurance. Also available at http://www.ncqa.org/Programs/HEDIS/. Accessed March 14, 2003.

[22] National Committee on Quality Assurance. The state of health care quality, 2002. Washington, DC: National Committee for Quality Assurance. Also available at http://www.ncqa.org/sohc2002/. Accessed June 7, 2003.

[23] Enthoven AC, Kronick R. A consumer-choice health plan for the 1990s. N Engl J Med 1989;320(2):94–101.

[24] Enthoven AC. The history and principles of managed competition. Health Aff (Millwood) 1993;12(Suppl):24–48.

[25] Maxwell J, Briscoe F, Davidson S, Eisen L, Robbins M, Temin P, et al. Managed competition in practice: "value purchasing" by fourteen employers. Health Aff (Millwood) 1998;17(3):216–26.

[26] Dubois RW, Brook RH, Rogers WH. Adjusted hospital death rates: a potential screen for quality of medical care. Am J Public Health 1987;77:1162–7.

[27] Lohr KN. Outcome measurement: concepts and questions. Inquiry 1988;25(1):37–50.

[28] Thomas JW, Hofer TP. Research evidence on the validity of risk-adjusted mortality rate as a measure of hospital quality of care. Med Care Res Rev 1998;55(4):371–404.

[29] Schauffler HH, Mordavsky JK. Consumer reports in health care: do they make a difference? Annu Rev Public Health 2001;22:69–89.

[30] Lieberman T. In search of quality health care. Consumer Reports 1998;63(10):35–40.

[31] Kassirer J. The use and abuse of practice profiles. N Engl J Med 1994;330:634–6.

[32] Hofer TP, Hayward RA, Greenfield S, Wagner EH, Kaplan SH, Manning WG. The unreliability of individual physician "report cards" for assessing the costs and quality of care of a chronic disease. JAMA 1999;281:2098–105.

[33] Kleinke JD. Release 0.0: clinical information technology in the real world. Health Aff (Millwood) 1998;17(6):23–38.

[34] Eisenberg JM. Doctors' decisions and the cost of medical care. Ann Arbor (MI): Health Administration Press; 1986.

[35] Davis DA, Thomson MA, Oxman AD, Haynes RB. Evidence for the effectiveness of CME: a review of 50 randomized controlled trials. JAMA 1992;268:1111–7.

[36] Davis DA, Thomson MA, Oxman AD, Haynes RB. Changing physician performance: a systematic review of the effect of continuing medical education strategies. JAMA 1995;274:700–5.

[37] Oxman A, Thomson M, Davis D, Haynes R. No magic bullets: a systematic review of the 102 trials and interventions to improve professional practice. Can Med Assoc J 1995; 153:1423–31.

[38] Davis D, O'Brien MAT, Freemantle N, Wolf FM, Mazmanian P, Taylor-Vaisey A. Impact of formal continuing medical education: do conferences, workshops, rounds, and other traditional continuing medical education activities change physician behavior or health care outcomes? JAMA 1999;282(9):867–74.

[39] Cabana MD, Rand CS, Powe NR, Wu AW, Wilson MH, Abboud PA, et al. Why don't physicians follow clinical practice guidelines? A framework for improvement. JAMA 1999;282:1456–65.

[40] Greco PJ, Eisenberg JM. Changing physicians' practices. N Engl J Med 1993; 329(17):1271–3.

[41] Soumerai SB, Avorn J. Principles of educational outreach ("academic detailing") to improve clinical decision making. JAMA 1990;263(4):549–56.

[42] Robinson JC. Theory and practice in the design of physician payment incentives. Milbank Q 2001;79(2):149–77.

[43] Wickizer TM, Lessler D. Utilization management: issues, effects, and future prospects. Annu Rev Public Health 2002;23:233–54.

[44] Wickizer TM, Lessler D. Do treatment restrictions imposed by utilization management increase the likelihood of readmission for psychiatric patients? Med Care 1998;36(6): 844–50.

[45] Wickizer TM, Lessler D, Boyd-Wickizer J. Effects of health care cost-containment programs on patterns of care and readmissions among children and adolescents. Am J Public Health 1999;89(9):1353–8.

[46] Lessler DS, Wickizer TM. The impact of utilization management on readmissions among patients with cardiovascular disease. Health Serv Res 2000;34(6):1315–29.

[47] Grol R. Beliefs and evidence in changing clinical practice. BMJ 1997;315:418–21.

[48] Grol R, Baker R, Moss F. Quality improvement research: understanding the science of change in health care. Quality and Safety in Health Care 2002;11(2):110–1.

[49] Wyszewianski L, Green LA. Strategies for changing clinicians' practice patterns: a new perspective. J Fam Pract 2000;49:461–4.

Address reprint requests to

Leon Wyszewianski, PhD
Department of Health Management and Policy
School of Public Health
University of Michigan
109 Observatory
Ann Arbor, MI 48109-2029

e-mail: leonw@umich.edu

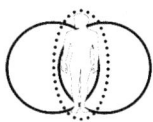
PROFESSIONAL AND PRACTICE MANAGEMENT SKILLS 1522–5720/03 $15.00 + .00

TEACHING SKILLS FOR PRACTICING PHYSICIANS

Neal Whitman, EdD and Thomas L. Schwenk, MD

We represent two different disciplines—Adult Education and Family Medicine—that have in common a focus on relationships, mentoring, and communication. These common interests guide this article on teaching skills. Our assumption is that although you may not be a faculty member whose career is devoted to teaching, you nevertheless have a commitment to teaching and would like to do it well. To begin with, every one of your patient encounters includes some form of teaching—after all, the Latin root of the word doctor is *docere*, to teach. In addition to teaching your patients, you instruct your office staff in new skills and you share knowledge with colleagues in your practice and on your hospital medical staff. Finally, some of you may precept medical students and residents who rotate in your practice.

This article offers seven lessons that we have learned in our professional lives. Our goal is to reinforce lessons about education that you have learned naturally in your professional life while observing good (to be emulated) and bad (to be avoided) teaching.

LESSON 1. THE MAGICAL NUMBER SEVEN (PLUS OR MINUS TWO)

We have a confession to make. Too much educational research is aimed at producing statistically significant results about trivial matters. Although this problem is well recognized and efforts are under way to improve this state of affairs [1], we are not apologetic about offering a finding of an educational research review published nearly 50 years ago by Harvard professor George A. Miller [2]. What Miller enunciates in this classic article is that the number of "chunks" of information that an adult can take in at

From the Department of Family and Preventive Medicine, University of Utah School of Medicine, Salt Lake City, Utah (NW); and the Department of Family Medicine, University of Michigan Medical School, Ann Arbor, Michigan (TLS)

one time and immediately recall is seven. Because some learners can handle nine (one standard deviation above the norm) and others only five (one standard deviation below the norm), Miller [2] succinctly sums up this finding in the title to his article: *"The Magical Number Seven, Plus or Minus Two: Some Limits on Our Capacity for Processing Information."*

We recommend that you use the "magical number seven" to guide your educational sessions. Of course, learners remember more when told less; therefore, in an informal session with patients or staff, you might want to highlight two or three key points. In a more formal session—for example, a talk at an annual family practice "update" or at an invited medical school lecture—you could organize the lecture around seven key points. This does not mean that you must limit the lecture to seven facts. Each of the seven key points, itself, could contain seven "bits" of information. Again, this is the Miller concept of "chunking" information.

When too much information is given at once, less will be retained. One study [3] showed that when patients were told eight facts they remembered only four. The "less is more" lesson also has been confirmed in studies of medical students [4]. Medical teachers who resist this educational lesson tell us, "But I have to cover all the material!" Our response is, "Don't you want to uncover it"? In 1925, Abraham Flexner [5], reflecting on his famous 1910 report on medical education, advocated that the medical teacher should aspire to be a "textbook with personality." Today, we live in an age of information overload. Because so much information is available to patients, staff, and students in print and electronically, we recommend that you prioritize what adults truly need to know. Your job is to make it memorable and understandable, not exhaustive (or exhausting!).

Our aim throughout this article is to make what we teach consistent with how we teach it: a principle known as "educational congruence" [6]. In the spirit of "practicing what we preach," here are seven tips to help you convey information to patients, staff, students, and colleagues.

1. Give the most important information first. If you begin with tangential facts, those are what will be remembered. Also, label the most important facts as such.
2. Use "advanced organizers"—in other words, preview the main subheadings of your message and review them along the way. We credit military trainers for the sound advice to "tell 'em what you're gonna tell 'em, tell 'em, and then tell 'em what you told 'em."
3. Avoid jargon. Using overly technical terms can create a problem for patients and medical students. Patients may be too shy to let you know that they do not understand, and students may be too embarrassed.
4. Use repetition for emphasis. Repeating information, directives, and assignments reinforces what is important to remember.
5. Check for understanding. Ask the listener to tell you in his or her own words what you have said. This technique aids in future recall and, at the same time, helps you to assess whether the material was grasped.

6. Make instructions specific, behavioral, and measurable. Your learner must leave the interaction knowing exactly what you expect to be done with the information.
7. When possible, include alternatives. Patients and students do well when given some choices in their instructions. Increased feelings of control and involvement markedly increase learning.

Giving information is a kind of "prescribing" (although you do not need a license to do so) and it can be as powerful (although usually not as dangerous!) as a class II drug. Physicians frequently give information to patients about preventing disease or about the features and consequences of the medical problem that brought the patient into the office. That power extends to staff and students. To be optimally effective, heed the warning of a plenary speaker who said that overdosing on facts is like giving thyroxine to a tadpole: one gets an "instant frog," but unfortunately a rather small one [7]. Applying the magical number seven and using the seven tips offered here will turn your teaching into potent medicine.

LESSON 2. MIND THE GAP

We are not recommending that you shop at the Gap store. We are playing on the announcements and signs found in the London Underground, which refer to the space between subway cars and the edge of the platform. "Mind the Gap" is the British version of "Watch Your Step," reminding travelers to use caution when entering or leaving the train. We recommend that, in your teaching role, you "mind the gap" or space between where learners are and where you want them to be or, even more powerfully, where they want to be.

When you mind the gap as a teacher, you assess the learner's needs, just as a physician diagnoses a patient's needs. In other words, before you treat a patient, you define the problem that warrants your intervention and correction. Likewise, before you instruct patients, staff, or students, you should define their educational needs. We could call this process "educational diagnosis." The term traditionally used by educators is "assessment," which literally means "to sit beside" or "to assist the judge" [8].

Harkening back to the patient analogy, we acknowledge that sometimes family physicians must treat without a definitive diagnosis. Likewise, there are times when physician teachers must and should instruct in the absence of a full-blown needs assessment. Nevertheless, there should be some notion of a gap in knowledge, attitudes, or skills before you begin to teach.

You want to share knowledge that is on target. You do not want to convey information that the learner already possesses—which would be a waste of time—nor do you want to neglect what the learner does not know, but needs to know. The watchword here is "need to know," not "nice to know."

You want to shape attitudes based on values and beliefs that you believe are essential to patient, staff member, or student growth and development.

You want to sharpen skills based on some measure of what the learner can and cannot do. In this way, you can build on existing skills; correct bad habits; and, when necessary, start from scratch.

So, how do you assess the existing knowledge, attitudes, and skills? Begin by asking! You will find that, just as some patients are insightful about their medical diagnosis, your learners may be insightful about their educational needs. Of course, not all patients are insightful. In medical practice, you most likely unconsciously have used a precept emphasized in kindergarten when you were taught how to cross the street: Stop, Look, and Listen. By the same token, Stop, Look, and Listen to your patients, staff, and students. Evaluate how well they know and understand their own needs. If they are insightful, then follow the direction they give you. If they appear less than insightful, that in itself is important information. Start where they are and aim your first instructional efforts at finding common ground.

To mind the gap, it is most helpful to involve patients, staff, and students in their own needs assessment. As noted by Leland Bradford [9], the cofounder of the National Training Laboratory, "It is ineffective for someone else to make the diagnosis for the learner—a frequent fault in education." Thus, we recommend that you take into account the learner's motivations, desires, anxieties, insecurities, and perceptions. Remember that the assessment of learners, like the diagnosis of patients, is a two-way process.

LESSON 3. IT'S ABOUT TIME: USING TIME WISELY

Time may or may not be a problem; it depends on where you are teaching. When you teach a hospitalized patient, you have a "captive" learner—he or she is not going anywhere fast! In your office, both you and the patient can hear the clock ticking, so your instruction needs to be succinct and efficient. Likewise, when supervising students and residents in the hospital, you and they have considerable control over the time required to accomplish both patient care and teaching objectives. In your office, however, patients are available for a very short time, and usually there is another patient ready to be seen. Despite the many interesting points yet to be made about the first patient, you have to move things along [10].

Ambulatory teaching also is characterized by the need to be prepared without having the time required to prepare. The range of potential patients, problems, and teaching points is large; the predictability of which problems and teaching points are most relevant is minimal; and there is not enough time to address adequately all possible interesting and valuable teaching objectives. Ambulatory teaching occurs in somewhat of a crisis milieu, in which the teacher always must make choices about how to use the precious, limited, and usually inadequate time available for multiple, competing objectives.

So, what is the teacher to do?

Teachers and learners often are dealing with different emotional stresses and professional objectives. Teachers are hoping that all of their teaching encounters will be exciting, effective and memorable, whereas learners usually are thinking more about survival—that is, they are worried about their patient care responsibilities, anxious about their personal lives, concerned with whether the teacher is interested in their growth and learning, worried about whether they know enough to impress the teacher, and thinking about how hard their upcoming night on call will be. Teachers would do well to take these considerations into account when planning their work, making decisions about teaching objectives, setting priorities for the use of precious time, and accepting that, as Mark Twain has said, "wisdom is like a watch—you don't have to tell everyone what time it is."

Here are some strategies to help you make the best use of the precious teaching time you have.

> Whenever possible, take time at the beginning of a clinic session to preview with the student or resident the patients to be seen. Consider how the learner might be involved best, if at all; remember that not all patients need to be or probably should be seen by a medical student. Focus in particular on any office protocols, past encounters that might be relevant, or specific objectives to be addressed with a particular patient. In a similar fashion, you can preview the learner's needs, prior experience, and learning objectives, and match those with the clinical goals for a specific patient. This assessment and preview will lead naturally to a rapid negotiation of agendas and objectives—for a specific patient encounter, for a clinic session together, or for the entire clerkship rotation. Such a negotiation and explicit discussion of objectives will help you make better and faster decisions about what to teach and how to teach it.
>
> Use your precious teaching time to emphasize concepts, analysis, synthesis, and generalizability rather than facts and memorization. The transmission and retention of facts is better done at another time with other methods. The value of personal contact between the teacher and learner is to focus on the well-known dilemma that "life is the art of drawing sufficient conclusions from insufficient premises." The assessment of the value and quality of clinical data, its contribution to clinical decision making, the consequences of such decision making, and a sensitivity analysis regarding hypothetic scenarios all are far more important ways to use precious time than is simply reciting facts for the learner to remember. This approach will lead to the frequent use of the following questions in your interactions with learners:
>
> "What do you think is going on?"
>
> "Why?"
>
> "What if...?" (using a wide range of hypothetic changes in the clinical data as they are gathered by the learner; eg, by varying the patient's age, the absence of a particular test, or a different test result).

"In general..." (making more general points about either the specific patient being discussed or about the teaching points revealed).

"In this particular case...".

"In the future..." (emphasizing what you most want the learner to remember about this encounter, recognizing that there are many choices for this teaching point).

Organize your interactions with the learner according to the Micro-skills Teaching Model developed by Neher et al [11]. Having a relatively standard approach to most encounters will help you make the most of the precious time.

Get a commitment—push the learner to organize his or her thoughts in a clear assessment, provide some tentative commitment to a diagnosis and plan, and exhibit a willingness to engage in some discussion of a plan in which he or she has some investment.

Probe for evidence—do not accept assessments and conclusions at face value, even when apparently insightful and correct, but push beyond the assessment to an understanding of how the learner made the assessment.

Teach general rules, reinforcing the questions described above.

Reinforce what was done correctly; that is, give positive feedback for good performance and correct mistakes when need be. (More information about giving feedback is provided in lesson 5.)

Finally, to these behaviors we also would add that most teaching encounters (eg, a half-day in clinic together) should conclude with an independent study assignment—that is, a follow-up activity that expands on the patients discussed and issues raised. It sometimes is helpful to tell the student to remind you of such an assignment at your next meeting, so that the student has the opportunity to demonstrate his or her follow-through and to receive credit for doing what you asked. Some of the best questions or topics for such independent study will arise from questions that come up in the middle of a busy clinic session. You can "bookmark" these topics by noting that they deserve some additional discussion later, when there is more time, and that the student should remember to ask about them at the end of the day.

LESSON 4. PROFESSIONAL INTIMACY, ROLE MODELING, AND MENTORING

The teacher–learner relationship is a more intense, emotional, intimate relationship than either teachers or learners perceive. As a clinician, you already are sensitive to the fact that in the physician–patient relationship, information is transmitted, not for its own sake, but for the sake of behavioral change. Likewise, when teaching staff and students, your aim is that they will do something new or different as a result of the interaction. Thus, whether you are interacting with patients, staff, or students, tension is inevitable. Why? Because you are asking your "learners" to "unlearn" something that they previously thought to be true, to behave differently, to think differently, or to view a problem or procedure differently because of your opinions and influence. This tension ultimately is a matter of ego threat; teachers are, in a sense, invading the learner's emotional space and threatening ideas and beliefs previously held to be true.

The teacher can overcome learner resistance to change by building trust. You would do well to keep the need for trust in mind at all times during your interaction with learners, in whatever setting—whether in a large or small group, during a brief encounter or in a longer relationship, and whether dealing with seemingly minor teaching points or with some significant interpersonal confrontation. It may be that there is little tension, that the learner is receptive, and that the issues are relatively low threat. However, it may help to assume that what you are asking the learner to do is going to be met with some resistance and therefore will require some trust on the part of the learner to accept your teaching and feedback constructively (see lesson 5 for more information about feedback).

The need to build trust leads to several aphorisms that may help you. (The attributions are somewhat unclear, but all are commonly cited among professional educators.)

> "Students don't care how much you know until they know how much you care."
> "Influence students to be independent of your influence."
> "Teaching is the art of creating within others the desire to help themselves."

With regard to the more specific role of mentoring—which is a defined, intense, and long-term teaching responsibility—there are certain characteristics of successful mentors that are relatively universal, irrespective of the level or domain of the mentor–protégé relationship [12]. The successful mentor

> Has a high level of personal accessibility.
> Has excellent communication skills.
> Avoids abusive relationships and interactions.
> Offers specific advice about goals, resources, tactics, and means.
> Gives specific advice about and provides access to activities, contacts, opportunities, and assignments that can further the protégé's career.
> Separates professional versus personal decisions (with a bias toward the former and away from the latter, unless specifically requested, while remaining within appropriate boundaries).

The reality of even the best mentor–protégé relationship is that there is the potential for abuse of the protégé by the mentor, often unintentionally, because the mentor is filled with enthusiasm for the many opportunities and possibilities that he or she could provide to the protégé. Often the successful mentor eventually is rejected by the successful protégé. This is, to some extent, an expected and natural outcome of the protégé's growth and success; however, it often leads to a sense of failure by the mentor and of loss by the protégé.

In conclusion, we recommend that you create professional intimacy with all of your patients, staff, and students so that you can effect change successfully. When you create professional intimacy, you will find that some patients, staff, and students may select you as a role model, so choose your words and actions carefully—you never know when you are being watched and emulated. Finally, in special cases, you may become a mentor. When mentoring, despite the potential disadvantages and risks, the relationship between you and your protégé can be one of great satisfaction, effectiveness, and emotion, rivaling that of parent and child. Professional intimacy, role modeling, and mentoring all have the same goal: to help another person grow and develop while becoming less dependent on you.

LESSON 5. GIVING AND RECEIVING FEEDBACK

Feedback is information about current performance designed to improve performance in the future. It can be positive, because current performance is good and you want to see more of it or it can be negative, because current performance is not good and you want to see it changed. It is understandable that your patients, staff, and students will not like negative feedback because, no matter how tactful you are at giving it, most people like to think of themselves as competent and successful. Also, negative feedback hurts more when it comes from someone who is highly respected (in this case, you).

Despite how difficult it is for "learners" to receive it, feedback is a critical domain of successful teaching. Here are some pointers on how to give feedback successfully [13]:

- Be as specific as possible, using examples and making reference to actual behaviors observed. When negative feedback is too general, it deteriorates into criticism; when positive feedback is too general, it becomes a compliment—fun to get, but not influencing future behavior.
- Focus on things that can be changed, with careful attention to those things that are most critical to the learner's eventual success. If you comment on a trait ("You're insensitive!"), your learner does not know how to improve performance. By focusing instead on a behavior ("You need to listen before you talk."), the learner then will know what to do.
- Give positive feedback only when deserved. Nonessential kudos will dilute the impact when important behavior is observed and noted. If every encounter is praised ("Nice smile!"), you run the risk that your patient, staff member, or student will not pay attention when it truly counts.
- Avoid abusive behavior. When you do need to be critical, there is no reason to be demeaning or belittling. You are commenting on the

patient, staff member, or student's behavior, not his or her personal worth.

- Consider your timing. When possible, give feedback immediately after you have observed a good or bad behavior. However, this is not always possible, and may not be desirable! When you decide to delay your feedback, use the "bookmark" method of letting the learner know that you would like to discuss a specific event or incident later in the day when there is time. This will "mark" the situation in the learner's mind so that subsequent discussions are more effective.
- Start your feedback session listening to the learner. The best feedback often is learner generated. Especially with a learner with whom you have spent considerable time, your request for self-evaluation will help you to modify and complement your own observations. Keep in mind, however, that your learners (especially medical students) will likely be harder on themselves than you would be.
- End your feedback session again with the learner. Check for understanding by asking your patient, staff member, or student to paraphrase the substance of your comments. This will let you know whether your learner has grasped the essence of your feedback.

Whenever you give feedback, it is important to teach learners how to evaluate their own progress. Your feedback is very helpful along the way, but, at the end of the day, patients, staff, and students must learn to gauge their own progress because you have not "signed on" to look over their shoulders for the rest of their lives.

Finally, an important aspect of feedback is the opportunity it gives you to role model an important two-way interaction. To accomplish this, occasionally ask the learner to give you feedback about your teaching skills. By being gracious about the positive and mature about the negative, your patients, staff, and students will learn a professional and constructive approach to both giving and receiving feedback.

LESSION 6. OPTIMAL STRESS IN TEACHING AND LEARNING

Stress, as you know from personal experience, is a normal part of everyday life. Taking your own "stress pulse," you probably have noticed that sometimes it is a good thing—a little pressure can be motivating. On the other hand, too much of a "good thing," is simply that: too much. When you feel too much pressure, which can be thought of as "distress," your performance may suffer. This observation is consistent with a key educational principle confirmed by research: people learn best when there is an optimal level of stress: not too much and not too little. The effect of stress on learning has been studied in animals and humans and the results are remarkable: there is a curvilinear relationship, in the form of an inverted U, between stress and learning. People learn less when there is too little stress (they do not feel challenged) or when there is too much stress (they feel threatened) [14].

The principle of optimal stress states that people learn best when they feel challenged, but not threatened. You probably have been making use of this key educational principle all along. Consider a patient with a new diagnosis of cancer. When your patient hears the word "cancer" for the first time, his or her mind shuts down. Due to your patient's distress, you minimize how much information you give in that initial interview, or you might be mindful that whatever information you do convey will have to be repeated at your next visit—and perhaps even the visit after that.

The optimal stress principle can serve you well in all patient education efforts and not just when giving bad news. Some patients will need a little push when you ask them to consider a lifestyle change. Others may need gentle coaxing before being asked to do more. Your dosing of stress levels has to be tailored to the individual because not everyone experiences the same event in the same way and not everyone responds to stress in the same way. However, you can count on this general rule: given two people with equal knowledge and skills, the one with the higher motivation will perform better under conditions that are optimally arousing.

A clinician has observed [15],

> We use multiple levels of clinical questions while seeing patients in the office, and the same applies for questions we ask of students and residents while teaching.... The teacher needs to keep the level of questions asked at an optimal stress level.... It is important to offer enough challenge to force students to think and learn (without being overly anxious) and yet to avoid frustrations by providing support when their knowledge is not yet at that level.

We recommend that when you teach anybody anything, you consciously should look for signs of frustration, which would tell you that there is not enough stress on the learner, and for signs of anxiety, which would tell you that there is too much stress. A professor of psychology and education summed up this modulating process: "If challenges are too high one gets frustrated, then worried, and eventually anxious. If challenges are too low relative to one's skills one gets too relaxed, then bored" [16].

Thus, when you are wearing your "educator's hat," look at your learner in the midst of the interaction. If you see signs of boredom, step up the pace; and if you see signs of anxiety, back off. Physicians who consciously use this approach are "reflective practitioners," which leads us to the seventh and last educational lesson in this article.

LESSON 7. MINDFUL PRACTICE: REFLECTION-IN-ACTION

Here are some lessons imparted by experienced clinicians. What do they have in common?

A family physician treating a patient with bronchitis says, "We have talked about your smoking before. Maybe now is not the right time for you to quit smoking, but how about trying it for 1 day before your follow-up visit and we can talk about how it went"?

A family practice preceptor who has seen a patient with "a suspicious mole" tells a first-year medical student shadowing him that he never tells a patient, "Oh, it's nothing," because he does not want the patient to feel he or she "wasted the doctor's time."

A hospice nurse tells a third-year medical student that when taking care of a cancer patient, she finds that she can never go wrong by asking first, "What's this like for you"?, and then listening to the patient's answer.

A visiting professor tells house staff that when she reviews a patient chart before entering the examination room, she senses her feet on the floor, takes a deep breath, and only then knocks. She says that this ritual helps her enter the room with an open mind to whatever may happen.

A veteran attending physician recalls that long ago when he was a medical student stumped by a patient's diagnosis, a chief resident told him, "Don't just do something. Stand there!"

What these scenarios have in common is the value of mindful practice in handling a routine task. As described by one of its proponents [17], a mindful practitioner attends, in a nonjudgmental way, to the mental and physical process of everyday tasks to act with clarity and insight.

Working on "automatic pilot" is an understandable response to the typical, busy day of a family physician. You may recall learning about the reflex arc in medical school, which explains why tapping the patella tendon elicits the knee jerk. Now that you are in medical practice, you find that the "reflex arc" gets you through the day! Ultimately, though, what makes a physician a true professional, rather than merely a technician, is the ability to "stop and think" about what he or she is doing. Schön [18] calls this "reflection-in-action"; that is, the ability to think about what you are doing while doing it.

Think about what you are doing when you teach. Be mindful that you are "doing it" in the first place. Whether a patient, staff member, student, resident, or colleague sits or stands before you, be aware that if there is (1) knowledge you want to share, (2) attitudes you want to shape, or (3) skills you want to sharpen, then you are, in fact, a teacher. As a mindful teacher, when you find yourself in this role you can take a deep breath, step outside yourself, take note, and observe yourself in action! Ask yourself, as you are interacting with this other person, "Who am I"?, "Why am I here"?, "What am I doing"?, and "What do I want to accomplish"?

- So, who are you? At this moment, you might reflect and be mindful that you are a teacher helping someone acquire new knowledge, attitudes, or skills. You might be mindful that this acquisition cannot be forced: you can lead a student to wonder, but you can't make him or her think!
- Why are you here? In this one moment in time, you might reflect and be mindful that in helping another person, help—like beauty—is in

the eyes of the beholder. So, have you asked how you can be of help or service?

- What are you doing? Are you acting in manner that gets the "learner" involved and open to new experience? Are you asking that person to reflect as you are doing—to stand back and think about the experience?
- What do you want to accomplish? You probably have certain educational objectives in mind. Also consider, however, the relationship you are building and the connections between you and the learner that occurred today that might lead to even higher levels of learning tomorrow.

Finally, after the educational experience is over, consider "reflection-after-action." That is, take a moment later that day to take a deep breath, step back, and ask yourself, "How did that go"?, "Was my approach effective or not"?, and "What, if anything, will I try differently in the future"? The truly outstanding teacher reflects in this fashion after every educational encounter, even when most are successful or even lauded.

Mindful practice and reflection-in-action already may be healthy habits you use in medical practice. We agree with one communication specialist who noted that physicians, by and large, are excellent listeners, but more so when interacting with patients than with others. The pitfall that some physicians face is that they do not use the same quality of mindful practice elsewhere as they do in the examination room [19]. Therefore, don't forget your staff, your students, and your colleagues—after all, don't they deserve the same attentive mind as your patients?

We hope that this last lesson is merely a reminder to use teaching skills already developed and used in other settings. For over 20 years, we have been reminding medical practitioners that they possess powerful communication skills that they use every day in providing patient care. Given an opportunity, a little guidance, and good intentions, physicians have the natural ability to become outstanding teachers.

SUMMARY

Family physicians have many opportunities to teach their patients, staff, and colleagues. Some physicians also precept medical students and residents in their offices. All these "learners" in a physician's life will benefit if the physician allows the seven lessons offered in this article to guide his or her educational practice.

Key points

- Less is more. Focusing on a few critical learning objectives accomplished well is better than covering too much material superficially.

- Let learners "diagnose" their own needs. Your role is to help them meet the learning objectives they have defined and support them as they carry out their learning plans.
- Time is precious. Especially in an office setting, be aggressive in managing this time for the benefit of the learner and the patient.
- Establish a strong and positive relationship with your learners. Be professionally intimate with all, realize that you will be a role model to some, and be open to the possibility that you may mentor a few.
- Give both positive and negative feedback. Establish an environment in which mistakes are expected and are viewed as learning opportunities, not permanent failures.
- Titrate the stress of the learning environment. Optimal learning does not occur at extremely low or extremely high levels of stress, but rather at a middle level that is enough to provide focus and energize the learner without causing boredom or paralysis.
- Be mindful. The best teachers are those who continue to learn from their own experience—both their successes and their failures. Constantly reflect, even as you are teaching, on how you are doing and how you can improve.

References

[1] Whitcomb ME. Research in medical education: what do we know about the link between what doctors are taught and what they do? Acad Med 2002;77(11):1067–8.
[2] Miller GE. The magical number seven, plus or minus two: some limits on our capacity for processing information. Psychol Rev 1956;63(2):81–96.
[3] Kaufman DM. Applying educational theory in practice. BMJ 2003;326(January):213–6.
[4] Russell I, Hendricson WD, Herbert RJ. Effects of lecture density of medical student achievement. J Med Educ 1984;59(11):881–9.
[5] Flexner A. Medical education: a comparative study. New York: Macmillan; 1925.
[6] Whitman N. Notes of a medical educator. Salt Lake City (UT): University of Utah School of Medicine; 2001. p. 69–71.
[7] Smith L. Medical education for the 21st century. J Med Educ 1985;60(2):106–12.
[8] Anderson S, Ball S, Murphy RT. Encyclopedia of educational evaluation. San Francisco (CA): Jossey-Bass Publishers; 1977.
[9] Bradford L. The teaching-learning transaction. Adult Educ 1958;8(3):135–45.
[10] Woolliscroft JO, Schwenk TL. Teaching and learning medicine in the ambulatory setting. Acad Med 1989;64:644–8.
[11] Neher JO, Gordon KC, Meyer B, Stevens N. A five-step "microskills" model of clinical teaching. J Am Board Fam Pract 1992;5:419–24.
[12] Ramanan RA, Phillips RS, Davis RB, Silen W, Reede JY. Mentoring in medicine: keys to satisfaction. Am J Med 2002;112:336–41.
[13] Whitman N, Schwenk TL. The physician as teacher. Salt Lake City (UT): Whitman Associates; 1997.
[14] Whitman N, Spendlove D, Clark C. Student stress: effects and solutions. Washington (DC): Association for the Study of Higher Education; 1984.
[15] Benzie D. Levels of questioning for learners. Fam Med 1998;30(1):12–4.
[16] Czikszentmihaly M. Finding flow. New York: Basic Books; 1997.
[17] Epstein R. Mindful practice. JAMA 1999;282(9):833–9.
[18] Schön D. Educating the reflective practitioner. San Francisco (CA): Jossey-Bass Publishers; 1987.
[19] Wallace L. How can we listen more effectively to colleagues and staff? The Healthcare Collaborator 2003;3(4):6–10.

Further Readings

Parker PJ. Let your life speak. San Francisco (CA): Jossey-Bass, Publishers; 2000.
Paulman PM, Susman JL, Abboud CA. Precepting medical students in the office. Baltimore (MD): Johns Hopkins University Press; 2000.
Whitman N, Schwenk TL. The physician as teacher. 2nd edition. Salt Lake City (UT): Whitman Associates; 1997.
The residents' teaching skill website. Available at http://www.ucimc.netouch.com/ (an extensive Web site focused on resident teaching skills but applicable to all medical teaching and teachers, includes a detailed set of references and resources). Accessed October 18, 2003.

Address reprint request to

Thomas L. Schwenk, MD
Department of Family Medicine
L2003 Womens
Box 0239
Ann Arbor, MI 48109

e-mail: tschwenk@umich.edu

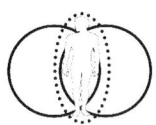
PROFESSIONAL AND PRACTICE MANAGEMENT SKILLS 1522–5720/03 $15.00 + .00

MANAGING ORGANIZATIONAL TRANSITIONS
TAKING THE CHANCE OUT OF CHANGE

R. Dale Lefever, PhD

Change takes place no matter what deters it…. There must be measured, laborious preparation for change to avoid chaos. —Plato

"In its most raw and destructive form, change is truly 'chaos'—a loss of control. When people in organizations initiate change or respond to it with adaptations that increase productivity, we call it innovation. But, how can change be harnessed to competitive advantage? And, how can 'chaos' be avoided" [1]? The purpose of this article is to provide to physicians who are responsible for the leadership of change in their organizations some specific guidelines for managing this important process and taking the chance out of change.

It must be recognized from the start that the status quo is not an option. Every organization either will change or be changed. Thus, one of the primary responsibilities of physicians in leadership is to serve either as the champion for intended change in such areas as practice guidelines, emphasizing evidence-based medicine, or helping the organization cope with externally mandated changes such as Health Plan Employer Data and Information Set or Health Insurance Portability and Accountability Act regulations for quality control and security, or responding to pressures from third-party payers. In any instance, the primary issue is not whether medical organizations and clinicians will experience change, but only how well the change will be managed and whether the intended outcomes of the proposed change will be realized fully. It also is significant that the nature of the outcome has as much to do with how the change is managed as it does with the nature (content) of the change itself. As noted by Harry Levinson in an article by William Bridges [2], "the most critical problem

From the Department of Family Medicine, University of Michigan Health System, Ann Arbor, Michigan leaders have is that they don't understand the powerful impact of change on people. They are wise about the mechanics of change, but stupid about the dynamics of transition. That stupidity is dooming many of their change efforts to failure."

The content of this article presents a four-stage model to guide physicians in leadership through the process of managing a change, while keeping the overall organization functioning and maintaining its core values. The four stages to be described include:

1. Establishing the need, or clarifying the impetus, for the change.
2. Understanding and managing resistance to the change.
3. Confirming the vision and determining the organization's readiness to make the change.
4. Sustaining the change after initial implementation.

Although it is acknowledged that change does not move through these stages at an even or predictable pace, neither can any of these stages nor their order be ignored. Planning with these issues in mind, and using these categories to gauge where the organization is in the change process will increase the likelihood of a managed change initiative that achieves its intended purpose.

ESTABLISHING THE NEED, OR CLARIFYING THE IMPETUS, FOR THE CHANGE (STAGE ONE)

The first step in giving leadership to the change management process is to establish the intellectual basis for the proposed change itself. It is not enough that the leader feels and understands the need for the change. This need must be felt and understood by other key members of the organization and, particularly, by those most affected by the change. According to Kotter [3], the first failure in managing change is the failure to develop a sense of urgency across the organization. The challenge is to create a sense of urgency, "especially with respect to a crises, potential crises, or great opportunities to gain the aggressive cooperation of many individuals. The goal is to make the status quo seem more dangerous than launching into the unknown" [3].

To create a critical mass of understanding and sense of urgency regarding the need for the proposed change, it is essential that leaders confirm three key elements of the proposed change itself before moving forward with implementation. First, there must be clarification with regard to the *impetus* for the proposed change. The word impetus is being used in this context to describe who or what is disturbing the status quo. It is based on the concept of inertia, which is defined as the "tendency of an object at rest to remain at rest; or, if moving, to keep moving in the same direction, unless affected by some outside force" [14]. People simply want to know why they are being asked to change. In fact, a basic principle to be considered is that if people do not know why, the cost of change (for them) always will be too high.

The impetus for a given change either is from the external environment and mandated (eg, new federal or state law) and is designed to make the organization strategically more responsive to its constituents, or is from internal forces and voluntary (eg, the organization's own strategic plan) and is intended to achieve targeted organizational goals and objectives. It is important that everyone directly affected by the change understands who or what is driving the change and that both those driving the change and the change itself are considered to be legitimate. If the impetus for the change is regarded as inappropriate, illegal, or irrelevant, the change process will be difficult, if not impossible, to launch. All of the energy will go into thwarting the proposed change rather than seeking ways to adopt it either as given or in some modified form. Therefore, three fundamental questions need to be asked before initiating any change process: (1) Who presently feels and accepts the need to change?, (2) Who needs to feel and accept the need to change?, and (3) How widespread and shared across the organization is the need for the change? Kotter [3] suggests that as many as fifty percent of change efforts fail, due to the inability of the leadership to answer these types of questions.

Second, the *purpose* of the proposed change (ie, the benefits that the change is designed to produce) needs to be clarified. All change efforts should be goal oriented and initiated to meet the acknowledged needs of the organization and the people it serves. Thus, leaders should avoid fads and "pet projects" or the practice of simply making changes for change sake. If the purpose of the change is not clear, extra effort in implementation will not fill this intellectual vacuum. There needs to be a "legibility of purpose" from the start of the process or the integrity of the change will be compromised and resistance will be increased.

The other issue that compromises the integrity of the change process at the front end is the presentation of a secondary or more acceptable purpose to mask the true and less attractive primary purpose—for example, the promotion and enforcement of clinical guidelines by a Health Maintenance Organization under the guise of quality enhancement when cost savings form the primary motivations. Understandably, many people are skeptical of lofty goals that appear to be designed simply to achieve support, and fear that the related phenomena of the "hidden agenda" and the "slippery slope" really is at work. In these situations, the energy of the group goes into blocking the initiative before it gets started, based on the belief that once the change gains momentum it will be too late to stop it. A lack of candor with regard to the actual purpose of the change will cripple the process and destroy the credibility of the leadership proposing the change. As Duck [4] states,

> Organizations today are full of "change survivors," cynical people who have learned how to live through change programs without really changing at all. Their reaction is the opposite of commitment. They say things like, "I'll believe it when I see it," or, "Sure, this sounds great, but what happens when we don't make the numbers."

Ordinarily, any change is designed to achieve one or a combination of the goals of increasing the quality or quantity of the work performed, doing things more rapidly to increase productivity, or reducing costs by working more efficiently. All of these criteria for success are valid, but some may be less appealing than others. For example, an attempt to improve physician clinical productivity may be challenged on the grounds that it reduces the quality of care. Leaders should avoid the temptation for the "bait and switch" approach and opt for absolute candor about the purpose and intended benefits of the recommended change. Telling the truth about change is not an option. It also is the easiest thing to remember!

The third key element in establishing the intellectual basis for the change is to describe accurately *the content and scope of the change* (ie, what will be changed and who will be affected). The *content* of most changes is targeted to introduce new skills or procedures, to revise current structures, to develop new strategies, or to create a new organizational culture. Quite often, proponents of a change believe they are making a relatively small change in current skills or procedures, when they actually are modifying the organization at a higher level with respect to its structure, strategies, or culture. For example, the implementation of an electronic medical record in a practice affects the overall system far beyond simply eliminating the paper chart. It involves workflow analysis and redesign, physician and staff training, security, and even modifications to the facility.

The concept of *scope* relates to the proportion of the organization's purposes, procedures, and people that will be affected by the change. It is important to clarify the magnitude of the change up front so that people will know, in advance, which people, functions, and segments of the organization will be impacted. A small and circumscribed change is easier to manage than is one that will affect everyone at all levels of the organization. What often happens, however, is that leaders underestimate (intentionally or unintentionally) the full magnitude of the change proposed in an effort to get people to "buy in," and then have to manage the fallout when the true magnitude of the change becomes reality.

In summary, although the tendency in managing a change is to jump right into the process, any leader with high expectations for results needs to make sure that the above four issues of impetus, purpose, content, and scope have been clarified and are shared widely, in particular, by those who will be most involved and affected by the proposed change.

Together, the above four issues will determine the leadership requirements needed to manage the change process. For example, if the proposed change is externally driven and will touch the lives of everyone in the organization, the senior leadership probably will need to champion the change personally to give it full credibility, oversight, and support. If the change is internally driven and fairly circumscribed in scope (eg, the introduction of a new skill or procedure), the leadership responsibility probably can be delegated. The above four issues also will determine the amount of time required to present and gain acceptance for the change. Again, the larger the change in terms of scope and impact, the longer it will

---

Stage One Summary

Establishing the Need
Communicate the
- Impetus for the proposed change—who or what is disturbing the status quo?
- Purpose of the proposed change—who will benefit and how?
- Content of the proposed change—what new skills, procedures, structures, strategies, or cultures will be introduced?
- Scope of the proposed change—what purposes, people, or procedures of the organization will be involved most? How big is the proposed change with regard to its impact on people and the system?

---

take to introduce and integrate it into the current system. Finally, these four basic issues also provide guidance with regard to the amount of intergroup cooperation and coordination required to effectively manage the change. A major change that will alter the culture and cut across all major organizational boundaries will require significantly more coordination than does a change in the skill level of individuals in one unit within the organization.

UNDERSTANDING AND MANAGING RESISTANCE TO CHANGE (STAGE TWO)

Once the intellectual aspect of the need for the change has been addressed, the impact of the proposed change on people needs to be assessed carefully. In addressing these important issues, it must be understood that there is no direct cause-and-effect relationship between the idea being promoted and the reaction it will receive from those who are most affected.

This seeming paradox results from the fact that change is not a rational process. It is not irrational, but simply nonrational. People basically behave in ways that make sense to them, based on their values and on how they believe the proposed change will alter their current situation in the organization. This fact explains, at least partially, why many smokers continue to smoke, although they know the habit is unhealthy; why intelligent people refuse to wear seat belts; why patients decline to complete, or even fill, their prescriptions; and, why physicians fail to adopt healthy lifestyles. Simply stated, knowing and doing represent two distinct levels of behavior and the first is not predictive of the second. One comedian stated it well in the story of a couple who smoked and lost their dearly loved dog to cancer. The woman immediately stopped smoking and the man went out and bought a new dog. People respond individually and selectively to change.

This important reality should alert those who are leading change that innovations simply are not accepted on their merits and that data, in and of itself, is not likely to motivate people to the degree necessary to successfully implement the change. A good idea certainly is necessary, but it is insufficient to bring about meaningful change. In fact, it is not uncommon for people to acknowledge the objective need for the change, but be unable or unwilling to adjust personally to the new behaviors required of them. One of the most important concepts to understand in change management, therefore, is that agreement with the intellectual basis for a change does not guarantee its acceptance. As Dickson [5] states, "The belief that enhanced understanding will necessarily stir a nation or an organization to action is one of mankind's oldest illusions." The leader must understand the personal transitions required and legitimize, rather than minimize, the stress the change will place on the individuals affected. Sensitivity to this issue will be increased if early and thoughtful consideration is given to the core reasons for why people often resist change.

Feelings of Uncertainty (The Fear of the Unknown)

People know how the current system works, but can only imagine, or hear projections, as to what the new situation will be like. It is not that the current situation is perfect, but the concern is that things, if changed, could be worse. As one pundit of change stated, "If you think you have a problem now, wait until you have solved it" [5]. This concern gives rise to the situation in which people often will prefer a "bad" known to a "good" unknown. As Kotter [3] states, "Employees will not make sacrifices, even if they are unhappy with the status quo, unless they believe that useful change is possible."

In actuality, most people do not fear change, but rather fear what they perceive as the irreversibility of change. They are afraid that if the proposed change does not achieve its intended goals, it will not be possible to return things to the way they were and that enormous and irretrievable resources will have been consumed. To counter this legitimate concern, there must be a careful analysis of the inadequacy of the current situation and a clear picture of how things will work if the recommended change is implemented. Too often a change—such as the introduction of a new reimbursement or incentive model—is initiated out of frustration with the current situation, without a clear model for how things will operate in the future being conveyed simultaneously. As one manager stated, "Either senior managers don't know what is going on or they don't want to tell us. Whenever someone asks a question, the response is we don't know yet. If they don't know, then what the hell are they doing disrupting everyone's life?" [6].

Sense of Loss (The Impact of the Change on the Individual)

As noted poet Shel Silberstein states, "If you are an early bird you get up early. If you are a worm, you learn to sleep late." Consequently, the degree of perceived personal loss depends on what each person values and on what each person believes the effects of the change will be in relationship to these values. In the process of change, everyone listens to the same radio frequency (ie, WIFM—what's in it for me).

People typically fear losing status, power, position, resources (eg, parking spots), and even their jobs. The leader needs to respect this fundamental filter, be candid about the impact of the change on peoples' lives, and be ready to renegotiate new arrangements when required. Leaders also need to remember that things can and do change fast, but people do not.

Threats to Competence (Perceived Ability to Function Effectively in the New Situation)

Most, if not all, physicians draw a significant level of their self-esteem from performing their work in a competent and professional manner. A change, however, often requires them to learn new skills, assume new responsibilities, or perform their current work in a new and unfamiliar way, for which they feel inadequately prepared. The need to learn new technology—for example, the requirements necessary to enter data directly into a hospital information system or a new billing system—can challenge those who feel unprepared in these areas. The leader needs to be prepared to offer the education and training required to equip those affected by the change and be patient with the anxiety that learning a new skill can create, especially for those who have performed their current work well for a long time.

Altered Relationships (Changes in the Internal Social System)

Physicians directing the change often focus so intensely on the content of the proposed change that they overlook the consequences the change will have for existing and important personal relationships within the organization. If, as a result of the change, people will be rearranged into new teams, moved physically to new locations, or have new reporting relationships, the change could be very difficult for them to accept. For example, the merging of two practices with different staff and different philosophies of practice, or the attempt to move from a single specialty to a multispecialty practice will raise important and sensitive issues with regard to leadership roles and relationships, independent of the cost effectiveness of the changes. Consequently, the leader should be careful not to disturb important social relationships unless absolutely necessary or be extremely sensitive to the "grief" and sense of loss that people will feel over seeing long-term friendships disrupted, if this is not avoidable.

Those leading the change also need to be prepared for "bargaining" in situations in which efforts to hold on to valued relationships can be intense. Again, a person can support the organizational need for the change, but be resistant to its implementation due to the impact it might have on important relationships. For example, the transfer of a team nurse might be the best option for the practice, but be of great concern to the nurse and physician who have enjoyed a meaningful working relationship over the years.

Lack of Involvement in the Decision (Being Left Out of the Process)

No criticism of the change process is more prevalent then the complaint by those affected that they were never consulted or informed of the change. Even when people realize that they have no choice, they still believe they deserve to be told directly about the change by the leaders who are making the decision. Leaders should make sure that they do not rely on the "rumor mill" to inform people and always should consider that input by those most affected by the change could result in a higher-quality decision with regard to its implementation. It is important to separate the decision on whether to change from the decisions on how to change. Many important changes have failed to be implemented because information from those who would be affected either was ignored or never solicited.

It also is important to note that most people work on an implied or actual "contribution-compensation" contract with the organization, which the proposed change could be seen to disrupt. For example, adding medical students to a service for the first time or adding in-house call at another site easily could draw the response, "That's not what I signed on for." Strebel [7] refers to this as a personal compact and states,

> Employees and organizations have reciprocal obligations and mutual commit-ments, both stated and implied, that define their relationship. Those agree-ments are what I call personal compacts, and corporate change initiatives, whether proactive or reactive, alter their terms. Unless managers define new terms and persuade employees to accept them, it is unrealistic for managers to expect employees fully to buy into changes that alter the status quo.

The implication here is not that leaders should not go forward because others will have their lives altered. The point is for leaders to understand where and how such changes impact others and to at least be willing to enter into negotiations with regard to options for implementation. Democ-racy does not mean that everyone gets his or her way. It does espouse, however, that everyone should have his or her say. Leaders of change need to be firm about the purpose of the proposed change, but flexible with regard to a variety of methods for its implementation.

William Bridges [2] refers to this second stage of the change process as "disengagement"—a time during which people need to let go of the current situation before they can embrace the new situation proposed by the change. He states [2],

> People have to let go of the old situation and (what is more difficult) of the old identity that went with it. No one can begin a new role or have a new purpose if that person has not let go of the old role or purpose first. Whether

people are moved or promoted, out placed or reassigned, they have to let go of whom they were and where they have been if they are to make a successful transition. A great deal of what is called resistance to change is really difficulty with this stage of transition.

Leaders must understand that change is a process and not an event, which means that people need time to adjust and can absorb change only at a reasonable pace. This does not mean, however, that leaders of change should reduce their persistence just because people go through phases of acceptance. As one manager stated, "I let the people visit pity city once a week, but I don't allow them to move there" [4].

In summary, there are some axioms of the change process that leaders of change should note.

- First, always remember that there is a reason for why things operate the way they do and that it is important to understand the history of the issues involved. Was this issue addressed before? If so, what happened? Are the same people involved? If so, what was their previous stance on this issue? Why was the current system put in place and are any of the reasons for it still valid? Leaders need to understand that each problem solved introduces a new unsolved problem.
- Second, the status quo is dynamic. Leaders may not know how much people care about what they do and how they do it until they recommend changes in these areas. Only then, when people feel threatened for any of the reasons just discussed, will the dynamic nature of the status quo be revealed.
- Third, no matter how "bad" anything is, someone likes it that way. Change, like beauty, is in the "eye of the beholder" and those proposing the change must be able to look at the change through the lens of those most affected. A simple question such as, "How is this person or group benefiting from the situation as it now stands?" can begin to inform those who are leading the change as to where the transition might be most difficult for others.
- Fourth, the cost of change may outweigh the cost of leaving things alone. You can do harm, because there is nothing intrinsically valuable about change. Unless mandated, leaders have a moral responsibility not to disrupt people's lives without counting the cost. Every leader must evaluate the cost of change versus the cost of leaving things alone. In performing this "dialectic," a leader can compare the costs of change to the costs of supporting the current system.

CONFIRMING THE VISION AND DETERMINING THE ORGANIZATION'S READINESS TO CHANGE

Once the intellectual need for the change is established (ie, impetus, purpose, content, and scope) and the nature and locus of the resistance is

---

Stage Two Summary

Managing the Resistance
Acknowledge the
- Feelings of uncertainty—the fear of the unknown.
- Sense of loss—the personal perceptions of how things will be different.
- Threats to personal competence—each individual's appraisal of their ability to succeed in the new system.
- Altered relationships—the impact of the change on the existing social system.
- Lack of involvement in the decisions—the need for people to be a part of renegotiating their future and feeling a sense of ownership.

---

assessed (ie, the nature and extent of the transition for those most affected), the focus needs to shift to describing the new reality that the change advocates. People will find it hard to let go of the current situation until they know what it is they are expected to embrace in its place. Bridges [2] refers to this stage as the period of "disorientation," during which people are in limbo. They are convinced that things are about to change and have accepted this reality, but they do not know yet what the changes will be. He states [2],

> People have to go through the "neutral zone" between their old reality and a new reality that may still be very unclear. In this no-man's land in time, everything feels unreal. But it also is the time when the real reorientation that is at the heart of the transition is taking place. Thoreau wrote that "corn grows in the night," and the neutral zone is the nighttime of transition.

Peter Senge [8] notes that a clear vision is the product of a dynamic tension between the current reality and the preferred reality. He states [8], "Creative tension comes from seeing clearly where we want to be, our 'vision,' and telling the truth about where we are, our 'current reality.' The gap between the two generates a natural tension for change." His key point is that analysis alone will not motivate people, no matter how bad current reality is described to be, and that vision alone will not be sufficient, no matter how lofty and inspiring it might be. Senge [8] notes, "What we need to grasp is that the natural energy for changing reality comes from holding a picture of what might be that is more important to people than what is." In a similar manner, Kotter [3] states,

> In every successful transformation effort that I have seen, the guiding coalition develops a picture of the future that is relatively easy to communicate and appeals to customers, stockholders and employees. Without a sensible vision, a transformation effort easily can dissolve into a list of confusing and incompatible projects that can take the organization in the wrong direction or nowhere at all.

This creation of a new future must be marked, in particular, by the establishment of the advantages and benefits of the proposed change. The issue, however, is not the "absolute advantage," but, rather, the "relative advantage" (ie, how the proposed change will be better than the program or procedure it is designed to replace). The relative advantage needs to be substantial and not just cosmetic. The changes proposed to improve the quality of care, enhance market share, or increase physician compliance with new billing and coding standards need to be tied to a criteria for measuring such success, and be worth the additional effort to achieve it.

In the context of systems theory, the change also must solve and not simply shift the problem. For example, law enforcement has found that arresting narcotics dealers in the inner city simply transfers the crime center to the suburbs. Automobile company executives have learned that rebates offered to increase sales of this year's cars often come at the expense of sales of next year's model. In the medical world, the addition of evening clinics designed to increase patient volume actually may only shift daytime visits to the evening.

It also must be understood that any change in one area of a system will create changes elsewhere. The whole truly is greater than the sum of its parts, and any change made in one part will change the whole. Several examples illustrate this principle: the decision to participate in a managed care market may increase patient volume, but also may come at the cost of physician independence and patient selection of their providers; a patient who quits smoking only to gain weight may experience a loss of self-esteem that results in a return to smoking to handle the increased stress; a prescription medication goes off patent and becomes less available to those who need it, because the over-the-counter price is more than the previous co-payment; or an increase in the co-payment to reduce overuse and increase revenues actually may discourage those who need the care and result in greater costs later on. All of these are examples of what Senge [9] refers to as "compensating feedback: when well-intentioned interventions call forth responses from the system that offset the benefits of the intervention."

In support of a systems perspective on change as described above, Senge [9] states,

> We need to destroy the illusion that the world is created of separate, unrelated forces. When we break apart complex problems to make them more manageable, we lose our intrinsic sense of connection to a larger whole. Trying to reassemble the pieces of a problem is similar to trying to fit together the fragments of a broken mirror to see a true reflection.

Once there is a consensus with regard to the vision for the change, and realistic expectations with regard to what it is intended to produce, the focus naturally turns to an assessment of the organization's capabilities to actually achieve its intended goals. Even though the need to change has been established and the emotional adjustments of people have been expressed and acknowledged, the leader still must assess the timing for the change and how well positioned the organization is to implement the change proposed. In conducting this important assessment, several issues should be addressed.

Available Political Support (Building the Necessary Political Coalitions)

No organization operates in a vacuum. Internal to any medical organization are numerous units with separate functions that all need to come together in support of the proposed change. Externally, there are all of the stakeholders and regulatory groups that influence the options available for implementation. If there is inadequate political support—internally or externally—for the proposed change, it either will fail or move forward with grave consequences in the future. Leaders should be aggressive in building political partnerships with other affected organizations and be extremely careful about pushing a change through without such support. The question is not whether another group should have jurisdiction over the project, but do they. This is clearly a situation in which you can "win the battle and lose the war."

Leaders, therefore, should identify carefully the key individuals or groups, and assess their relative role in support of the project. For example, are these individuals opposed to the change and prepared to challenge it; simply willing to let it happen, but without active support; ready to help it happen; or committed to making it happen? Every change effort needs a champion and every champion of change needs to build a coalition of support. As Kotter [3] states,

> Major renewal programs often start with just one or two people. In cases of successful transformation efforts, the leadership coalition grows and grows over time. But whenever some minimum mass is not achieved early in the efforts nothing much worthwhile happens. And, in most successful cases, the coalition is always pretty powerful in terms of titles, information, expertise, reputations and relationships.

Adequate Financial Resources (Gaining the Economic Commitments)

Every organization is faced with legitimate needs that exceed available resources. The proposed change must have a priority for resources within the organization and likely will need to compete with resources committed to established programs. Too often those affected by the change are asked to personally support a change that the organization itself is not willing or able to support. Frequently, this is the result of "low balling" the originally proposed change to gain its acceptance only to have the real "sticker shock" revealed in the process. As mentioned above in the section on emotional adjustments, people fear the irreversibility of change, where so much money has been spent and so much ego has been invested that reversing the project is almost impossible. Leaders of change need to count the costs and accurately represent them. There is an old adage on change that says, "in the business of change friends disappear and enemies accumulate." The underestimation of the full costs of change, either intentionally through deception or unintentionally through ignorance, is a predictable cause of failure in any change effort.

Because there always will be competition for scarce resources, the leader should confirm the organization's willingness and ability to support the change economically and communicate the priority of the project to the broadest audience possible. Nothing is more discouraging to people than to learn well into the implementation stage of a change that the resources to support them really are not available—for example, holding physicians accountable to a higher standard of productivity without providing the staff support necessary to achieve the new benchmarks; or, as often occurs with the implementation of an electronic medical record, funding the software and hardware, but having no funds available to support the time of the project team who is assigned the responsibility for implementation.

Compatible Social Support (Managing the Cultural Conflicts)

It is common for a good and innovative idea to challenge long-standing traditions and customs. The leader should learn the history of the issue being addressed and the values and norms that support the current practices targeted for change. The best idea in the world will be seriously challenged if it conflicts with deeply held beliefs and values within the organization. It is wise to check with the organization's historians and "value brokers" to learn if and how the proposed change will threaten the organizational culture. Many changes can be possible technically, yet unacceptable socially. For example, patient visits per hour can be increased, but not without some concern for quality of care. Medical practices can be run efficiently by professional managers, but not without some stress on physician autonomy. Co-payments can be increased, but not without some concern about the affordability of care. In the medical culture, any change that threatens the core values of the primacy of the doctor–patient relationship or physician independence and control will likely encounter both individual and institutional resistance.

Necessary Technical Capability (Assessing Adequacy of Existing Personnel, Equipment, and Systems)

No organization can afford to commit all of its resources to any one specific change. The organization must continue to function while implementing the change. The leader, therefore, should assess carefully the number and type of people needed to successfully implement the change, the technology required, and how much support from other areas of the organization is available to assist with this specific change. Not only is it important for people to believe the change is the right thing to do, they also must be convinced the organization has the internal capacity to accomplish the change. The leader must consider what other changes in the organization will be required to support this change and recognize that any change in one part of the system likely will have implications for the entire system.

Once the assessment of the four factors listed above is complete, the decision can be made to proceed as planned, modify the plan in light of issues identified, or actually delay or cancel the plan to implement the change. The leader should not let ego push a change forward, which is likely to damage the organization in the process. In an effort to make an informed decision at this point, there are five basic characteristics of successful change to be considered. Even if there is no choice but to implement a change because it is externally mandated, these characteristics are useful to guide implementation.

First, as mentioned earlier, the proposed change must demonstrate *relative advantage*. In their classic work on the diffusion of innovations, Rogers and Shoemaker [10] state, "Relative advantage, in one sense, represents the intensity of the reward or punishment resulting from adoption of an innovation. This can involve the degree of economic profitability, low initial costs, lower perceived risks, a decrease in discomfort, a savings in time and effort or the immediacy of the reward." The critical issue is that the relative advantages marketed match the relative advantages most likely to occur. Promoting an idea as one that will save money when costs only will be shifted, or promoting an issue on the basis of quality when the gain is political are ill-advised strategies that will damage the integrity of both the leadership and the project.

The second consideration to review before implementation is the *compatibility* of the proposed change with the existing values, past experiences, and needs of the affected groups. As stated by Rogers and Shoemaker [10], "Compatibility ensures greater security and less risk to the receiver and makes the new idea more meaningful to him," or, as one pundit noted, "It is easier to ride a horse in the direction it is running." Leaders, therefore, need to be conscious of the local cultures within their organizations and the communities they serve, and be prepared for substantial resistance if the proposed change flies in the face of deeply held values.

The third element involves the *complexity* of the change itself, or "the degree to which an innovation is perceived as relatively difficult to understand and use" [10]. An innovation such as the electronic medical record might be quite complex in its design, but if it is perceived to be "user friendly" in its application, the response can be quite favorable. The main goal for leaders of change is to present the idea in a concise and readily understandably manner so that those required to use it or be involved with it can see its application clearly and fully.

The fourth and final characteristic of successful change is the ability to pilot test the idea before full implementation (ie, to give it a reality check). The technology that works at the vendor's site often does not perform with similar success in the user's office. Rogers and Shoemaker

[10] refer to this as "trialability" or the ability to try ideas on the installment plan. There are basically three reasons for conducting a pilot operation before introducing the change across the entire organization: (1) to serve as an experiment and prove technical feasibility to top management, (2) to serve as a credible demonstration model for other units in the organization, and (3) to slow the pace of change and allow people to adjust in an incremental fashion [11]. The critical issue for the leaders of a change with respect to pilot testing is the selection of the site and the individuals to be involved in the pilot. If a site and a group are selected that are atypical, the ability to generalize to full implementation will be discarded. If a site and a group are selected where there is great resistance, it will not be clear whether the idea or the implementation was the cause of the failure. "The solution, therefore, is to be clear about the purpose of the test—experimental or demonstration—and then to choose the site that best matches the need" [11].

INSTITUTIONALIZING THE CHANGE (STAGE FOUR)

The fourth and final stage of the change management process addresses the need to integrate the proposed change into the existing system on a routine basis. In reality, the most difficult challenge of managing change is not the ability to generate a good idea, or even to start its implementation. The major challenge is sustaining a change over time (anyone who has been on a diet or dedicated himself or herself to an exercise program can attest to this). This last stage, therefore, addresses how to manage the transition period between ending the current activities and having the new activities widely supported and firmly in place. In this regard, one should expect, and plan to manage, the situation in which things probably will get worse before they get better. It is in this transition period, when the "bugs" are being worked out, that the change is the most vulnerable and will need the most support from top leadership. Bridges [2] refers to this as the new beginning or realignment stage and states, "Difficulties with making new beginnings come not from a difficulty with beginnings per se, but from a difficulty with endings and the neutral zones."

Stage Three Summary

Confirming the Vision and Determining the Organization's Readiness to Change
Clarify the
- Relative advantages of the change—how it improves on the current system.
- Systems involved—the changes the proposed change will cause and the changes the proposed change will need to support it.
- Organizational readiness—the political, economic, social, and technical requirements and current capabilities in each area.

There are basically three reasons why people support the implementation of a change. The first is called *compliance*, which means that they do it only to gain a favorable reaction in an effort to solicit support for some other project they plan to introduce or to avoid a conflict that they do not believe they can win. Neither of these reactions speaks to their understanding of, nor support for, the proposed change. The second basis for supporting implementation involves *identification*, which includes peer pressure and seeking to maintain a positive relationship with the leadership driving the change. Again, it should be noted that this level of acceptance may reflect loyalty or even friendship, but does not necessarily reflect a deep understanding of the change itself. The third level of acceptance is *internalization*. At this level, the support is not based on fear or friendships, but on the belief that the change proposed has intrinsic rewards and is the right thing to do. Although there will be those in the organization at each of these levels, unless people are able to internalize the change, it likely will falter for lack of a critical mass of support. The following issues are critical during this final transition stage and, if applied, will guide leaders in moving toward the ultimate stage of internalization.

Adequate Education (Preparing Individuals and Groups for the New Behaviors)

For people to support the change, they have to understand the new behaviors well enough to perform them. This will require education, training, or, at least, orientation. Regardless of the sophistication of the new skill, procedure, or process, people will need direct guidance and supervision during the transition period to make the break with the old system and to feel comfortable with the new way of doing business. The leader should not put maximum energy into getting people to "buy in" to the change and then not support them during the actual implementation stage itself. This is a classic error with respect to technologic change in which hundreds of thousands of dollars are poured into new equipment with comparatively little resources provided toward training people how to use it. It is estimated, for example, that only about 10% to 15% of the capability of the technology purchased actually is used by those it was designed to help.

Broad Commitment (Gaining Consistent Performance Across the System)

It is highly probable that every change will be challenged at some time during the initial implementation period by influential people who refuse to cooperate. This is a difficult but important situation to manage. People want to be treated fairly in general, but in times of change, perceived fairness is the most critical value. Those most affected by the change want to see the "equity of sacrifice" at work.

If some have to cooperate only because they have no power to resist, then they will resent it. The leaders responsible for directing the implementation stage cannot run and hide. They need to be willing to confront those in power who refuse to cooperate and set the goal of consistent performance across the system. Two approaches to handling this situation are for those who are directing the change to model the new behavior personally whenever possible, and to initiate the change at the point in the organization where it is needed most and the benefits will be most clear. Ultimately, however, those who seek to sabotage the change through noncompliance will need to be confronted.

> One company began its transformation process with much publicity and actually made good progress. Then the change effort ground to a halt because the officer in charge of the company's largest division was allowed to undermine most of the new initiatives. He gave lip service to the process but did not change his behavior or encourage his managers to change [3].

Motivation and Rewards (Aligning the Resources of the Organization with the Desired Behaviors)

One of the common complaints during periods of change is the communication of "mixed messages." People are told that one thing is important, but the reward system seems to promote different or even counterproductive behaviors. The leader can gain a great deal of support for the change during the early period by affirming those who are cooperating with the change through the appropriate distribution of resources and rewards. The people who get the new equipment first are the ones that need it and not those with a higher status who want it. The people who get the additional staff support, the necessary training, and the adjustments in their work to accommodate their new role in support of the change are those who deserve and will benefit from such resources.

Communication and Feedback (Describing and Celebrating Progress)

There generally is substantial interest and focus on a change at the immediate point of implementation. People, if not enthusiastic, are often at least willing to give the new activity a chance to succeed. This "honeymoon" period, however, will not last forever. People will want and deserve to know whether the new system is working. The leader must provide this feedback and celebrate in instances in which success is being realized. For example, if new clinical guidelines are introduced to alter physician prescribing patterns, then feedback on whether changes in these desired behaviors have occurred needs to be reported. Similarly, if special education is introduced to improve billing and coding accuracy, then regular feedback from chart audits should be planned at the start as part of this intervention. Regardless of the situation, it is important to apply the

---

Stage Four Summary

Institutionalizing the Change
Provide the
- New skills required—invest in training and education consistent with the requirements.
- Enforcement needed—negotiate within parameters and set deadlines for compliance.
- Resources needed for implementation—align the rewards with the desired behaviors.
- Feedback to those most involved—compare the intended results with the actual accomplishments against the criteria established.

---

criteria that were established at the start of the project for measuring success. Many change advocates are surprised when they learn that what they consider to be a success is viewed by others as a failure. This discrepancy generally is a result of differing expectations (eg, cost reductions versus quality improvements) concerning the proposed benefits of the change. To avoid this occurrence, the purpose of the change and how success will be evaluated should be declared at the start and monitored and measured throughout the implementation stage.

> Real transformation takes time, and a renewal effort risks losing momentum if there are no short-term goals to meet and celebrate. Most people won't go on the long march unless they see compelling evidence within twelve to twenty-four months that the journey is producing expected results. Without short-term wins, too many people give up or actively join the ranks of those people who have been resisting change [3].

Quinn [12] refers to this strategy as logical incrementalism and states, "Such incrementalism is not muddling. It is a purposeful, effective, proactive management technique for improving and integrating both the analytical and behavioral aspects of strategy formulation." Karl Weick [13] explains, "The challenge in change is to start with controllable opportunities that will yield visible results." Basically, people are motivated by seeing progress and leaders need to show them exactly that.

SUMMARY

Adherence to the above four stages of the change management process and the related issues will not guarantee success, but it will greatly enhance it. Although there often will be unexpected consequences, a well-managed change process will reduce such contingencies and make them more manageable, if and when they do occur. Leaders need to remember that change is not an acute event, but a series of transitions. Many important changes have been reduced in effectiveness, or even destroyed, because the leadership did not attend to both the content of the change and the process by which it was introduced and managed. With attention to this process, a leader can take much of the chance out of change.

Key Points

- The "actual" rationale and relative advantages of the proposed change are the most predictive of successful implementation. If people do not know why, the cost always will be too high.
- Things change fast, but people do not. Change is an event, but the process required for people to cope with change is best understood as a series of transitions over time.
- Implementation is not the ultimate goal. The real test is the ability to integrate and sustain the intended change over time.

References

[1] Schoonover SC, Dalziel MM. Developing leadership for change. Management Review 1986;July:55–60.
[2] Bridges W. Managing transition: making the most of change. 2nd edition. Cambridge (MA): Peseus Books; 2003. p. 19–50.
[3] Kotter JP. Leading change: why transformation efforts fail. Harvard Business Review 1995;March–April:59–67.
[4] Duck JD. Managing change: the art of balancing. Harvard Business Review 1993; November–December:109–18.
[5] Dickson P. Rules to rue. From Abbott's admonitions to Zymurgy's law. Mainliner 1978;December:50–5.
[6] Tichy NM, Devanna MA. In: The transformational leader. New York: John Wiley & Sons, Inc. 1986. p. 3–33.
[7] Strebel P. Why do employees resist change? Harvard Business Review 1996;May–June:86–92.
[8] Senge PM. The leader's new work: building learning organizations. Sloan Management Review 1990;Fall:7–23.
[9] Senge PM. The fifth discipline: the art and practice of the learning organization. Currency Doubleday 1994;57–67.
[10] Rogers EM, Shoemaker FF. Communication of innovations. Free Press; 1971. p. 139–60.
[11] Leonard-Barton D, Kraus WA. Implementing new technology. Harvard Business Review 1985;November–December:102–10.
[12] Quinn JB. Strategic change: "logical incrementalism." Sloan Management Review 1989;Summer:45–60.
[13] Weick KE. Small wins. Redefining the scale of social problems. American Psychologist 1984;January:40–9.
[14] New World Webster's Dictionary. Montevideo, Mexico: The World Publishing Company; 1978. p. 719.

Address reprint requests to

R. Dale Lefever, PhD
Department of Family Medicine
University of Michigan Health System
1500 East Medical Drive
Ann Arbor, MI 48109-0239

e-mail: dlefever@med.umich.edu

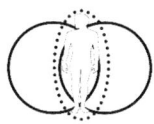

PROFESSIONAL AND PRACTICE MANAGEMENT SKILLS 1522–5720/03 $15.00 + .00

HEALTH BEHAVIOR MODELS: TOOLS FOR UNDERSTANDING AND FACILITATING PATIENT BEHAVIOR CHANGE

Rebecca A. Malouin, PhD, MPH

ROLE OF THE FAMILY PRACTICE PHYSICIAN

According to the American Academy of Family Physicians [1]

> Family practice is the medical specialty which provides continuing and comprehensive health care for the individual and family. It is the specialty in breadth which integrates the biological, clinical and behavioral sciences. The scope of family practice encompasses all ages, both sexes, each organ system and every disease entity.

The family physician is the initial point of contact to the health care system for many individuals. Responsible for "evaluating the patient's total health needs," the family physician is uniquely placed within a clinical context to evaluate and modify clinical and other factors affecting an individual's health status [1].

A survey of continuing medical education topics conducted in September 2002 indicated that approximately 23.8% of active members of the American Academy of Family Physicians rated the category of "health promotion/community health/prevention" a priority area and only 16.2% rated "health behavior change/risk factor reduction" as a priority area [2]. However, 7 of the 10 top causes of death in the United States are related to chronic disease [3]. Obesity is epidemic in the United States, with a corresponding projection of higher rates of chronic disease within the next century [4,5]. The promotion of healthy behaviors for prevention and

From the Epidemiology Services Division, Michigan Department of Community Health, Lansing, Michigan; the Department of Epidemiology, College of Human Medicine, Michigan State University, East Lansing, Michigan; and the School of Health and Human Services, Walden University, Minneapolis, Minnesota treatment of disease is imperative to reduce the burden of morbidity and mortality due to chronic disease in the United States. Mechanic [6] notes that

> As behavioral and chronic disease problems increasingly predominate with the aging of the population and changes in patterns of morbidity, the almost exclusive dependence on the diagnostic disease model may become less efficient in addressing the burden of illness and disability seen in primary medical care.

Family physicians are the initial contact to encourage healthier behaviors for many individuals, and health behavior models provide a broad context in which physicians can identify factors related to a patient's health status and health behavior.

DISEASE AND ILLNESS

Arthur Kleinman [7] distinguishes disease from illness. Disease is defined as an alteration in biologic structure or functioning, whereas illness is a patient's experience of the disease. Although disease encompasses a narrow biologic process, illness includes a patient's explanation for the distress caused by the pathophysiologic processes and the perception of, experience of, and response to symptoms and disability [7].

Although family physicians are trained rigorously to address disease, training in addressing illness, or a patient's experience of disease, often is left to other disciplines such as psychology or health education [8,9]. Furthermore, the limited contact that many physicians have with patients further reduces opportunities for discussion of nonclinical factors related to illness and disease [10,11]. As Kleinman [7] describes

> One unintended outcome of the modern transformation of the medical care system is that it does just about everything to drive the practitioner's attention away from the experience of illness. The system thereby contributes importantly to the alienation of the chronically ill from their professional caregivers and, paradoxically, to the relinquishment by the practitioner of that aspect of the healer's art that is most ancient, most powerful, and most existentially rewarding.

Health behavior models enable a physician to identify, with a patient, specific components of illness to better understand factors affecting illness and disease. By referring to commonly applied behavioral models in clinical practice, family physicians may quickly identify possible nonclinic factors associated with disease and possible intervention points most likely to affect behavior change.

HEALTH BEHAVIOR MODELS AS A TOOL

Health behavior models are operational tools developed from health behavior theories, used to provide a vehicle for understanding a health problem within a specific context. Models contain variables, or operational forms of elements of a theory. The most well-known behavioral models have been tested within a multitude of settings. However, not all models apply equally well in all settings [12].

Physicians can use behavioral models to identify factors affecting behavior that are not considered traditionally within a clinical setting [13]. Barriers and facilitators to a behavior, self-efficacy in performing a behavior, perceived severity of a health condition, and possible cues to action are examples of factors of which a physician may consider for inquiry during a patient consultation. Furthermore, the stage of change of the patient, from identification of personal risk to willingness and self-efficacy to take action, also is of interest in influencing behavior. Systematic collection of such information may reveal common factors in a patient population, and consequently, suggest subpopulation-level or population-level interventions.

EXAMPLES OF MODELS OR THEORIES

Models often are defined by unit of intervention, often characterized by individual, interpersonal, community, and multiple levels (Box 1). Models focusing on the individual and interpersonal would seemingly be the most useful for family physicians in clinical practice, due to the interpersonal nature of the physician–patient interaction. Individual-level models are particularly effective in identifying individual-level factors influencing behavior and identifying areas for effective counseling by a physician. Consequently, examples of individual-level models, including both static and stage-based models, are presented.

EXAMPLE OF A STATIC MODEL: THE HEALTH BELIEF MODEL

The Health Belief Model was developed in the 1950s by physicians in the US Public Health Service as a method for understanding factors associated with participation in screening programs for tuberculosis (Fig. 1) [14]. The model includes factors associated with behavior change and behavior maintenance. Individual perceptions, such as perceived susceptibility to and severity of disease; modifying factors, such as demographic characteristics, perceived threat of disease, and cues to action; and perceived benefits and barriers, each can influence the likelihood of a behavior change.

Use of the Health Belief Model at the Individual Level

Consider the following case: A 50-year-old man presents to a family physician with complaints about hypertension. He has read brochures about hypertension and has tried to reduce his stress through exercise, but does not feel he will be able to change his diet, especially reducing his salt

---

Box 1. Examples of health behavior models and theories by level of intervention

Individual

Static models
Health Belief Model
Theory of Reasoned Action and Theory of Planned Behavior

Stage-based models
Transtheoretical Model and Stages of Change
The Precaution Adoption Process Model

Intrapersonal
Social Cognitive Theory
Models of Social Networks and Social Support
Transactional Model of Stress and Coping
Interdependence Theory/Model of Social Influence and Interpersonal
    Communication

Community
Community Organization and Community-Building Practice
Diffusion of Innovations
Theories of Organizational Change
Communication Theories

Multilevel
Precede-Proceed Model
Ecologic Model

---

intake. In reviewing the components of the Health Belief Model, a physician may consider inquiring about barriers to, and the patient's perceived self-efficacy in, behavior modification.

Upon further questioning, the physician finds that due to his busy schedule, the patient often orders fast food on his way home from work or buys frozen foods that he microwaves for meals. Therefore, both the barrier of time and self-efficacy in selecting reduced-salt foods may be negatively influencing his intention to prevent hypertension. A family physician may intervene by encouraging a modification in diet and recommending a nutritional consultation.

Use of the Health Belief Model at the Population Level

A study in Vancouver, Canada [15], evaluated the association between subjective and objective factors in the determination of self-care in over 794 adults age 50 and over, diagnosed with one of three chronic diseases including arthritis or rheumatism, heart problems, or hypertension. Self-care was defined by 16 possible actions such as stress reduction,

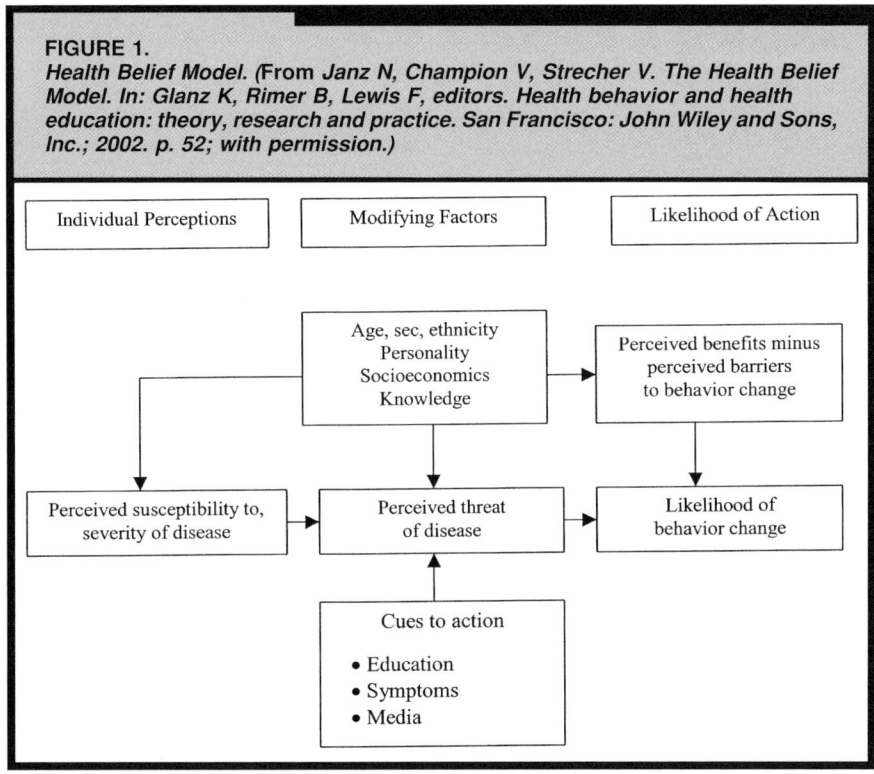

FIGURE 1.
Health Belief Model. (From Janz N, Champion V, Strecher V. The Health Belief Model. In: Glanz K, Rimer B, Lewis F, editors. Health behavior and health education: theory, research and practice. San Francisco: John Wiley and Sons, Inc.; 2002. p. 52; with permission.)

medication, reduced salt intake, reading about illness, consulting friends, and reduced smoking. Using the Health Belief Model as a framework for the selection of predictors of self-care, the investigators found that objective health care indicators (such as number of recent visits to a physician) were more important in predicting self-care behaviors engaged by older adults diagnosed with arthritis, whereas subjective indicators (such as self-efficacy and well-being) predicted self-care behaviors in those adults with heart problems and hypertension. The investigators [15] concluded, "Understanding self-care among older adults coping with chronic conditions is dependent on important dimensions of the illness context, in particular, the specifics of symptomology."

EXAMPLE OF A STAGE-BASED MODEL: THE TRANSTHEORETICAL MODEL

The Transtheoretical Model and Stages of Change, developed by Prochaska et al [16], provides a method of assessing the current and future

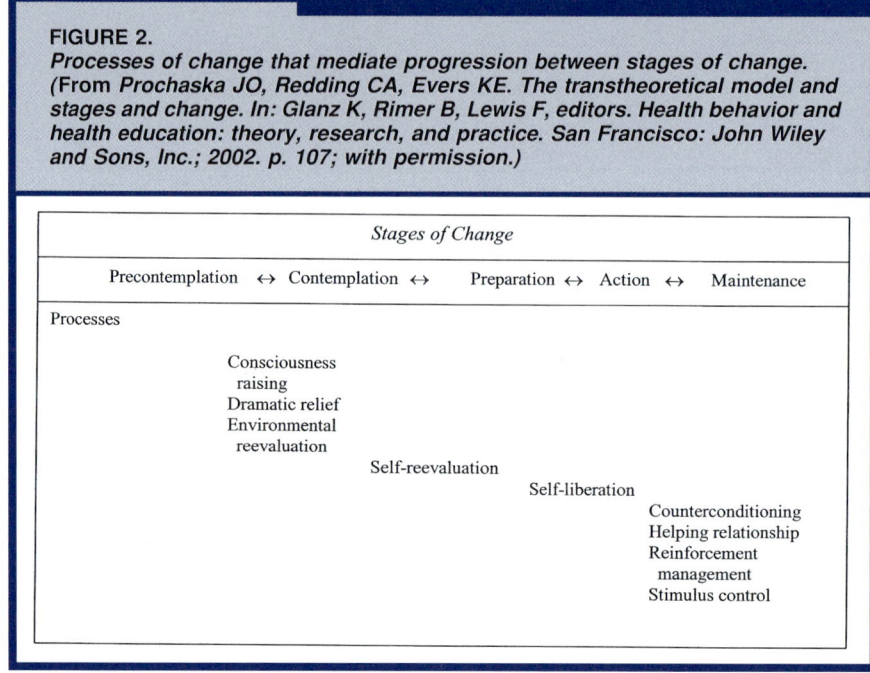

FIGURE 2.
Processes of change that mediate progression between stages of change.
(From Prochaska JO, Redding CA, Evers KE. The transtheoretical model and
stages and change. In: Glanz K, Rimer B, Lewis F, editors. Health behavior and
health education: theory, research, and practice. San Francisco: John Wiley
and Sons, Inc.; 2002. p. 107; with permission.)

stage of an individual or population on a continuum of stages of behavior change (Fig. 2). The stages of change include:

1. Precontemplation: No intention of change in behavior within the next 6 months.
2. Contemplation: Intention of change in behavior within next 6 months.
3. Preparation: Intention to change behavior in next month and has already begun steps to change.
4. Action: Has changed behavior for less than 6 months.
5. Maintenance: Has changed behavior for more than 6 months.

Mediators of the processes of shifting between stages include an individual's decisional balance between the benefits and costs of changing behavior and an individual's self efficacy in performing the behavior and avoiding unhealthy behaviors. Examples of processes of shifting between stages include consciousness raising, or collecting information about the behavior; self-liberation, or committing to the behavior change; and social liberation, realizing that social norms support the behavior [16].

Use of the Transtheoretical Model At the Individual Level

A 45-year-old woman with diabetes mellitus is seen by her family physician and is found to have a hemoglobin A_{1c} of 12%. Although counseled on the risks for diabetic complications with such an elevated hemoglobin A_{1c} during her previous clinic visit 1 year ago, she has not yet modified her lifestyle. In this case, according to the Stages of Change in the Transtheoretical Model, perhaps during her last visit she was in the precontemplation stage of change. Upon asking her whether she would consider modifications in her diabetes management, she indicates that within the next month she would like to begin lifestyle changes to reduce her risk of developing complications. According to the Transtheoretical Model, her physician may consider focusing on encouraging her decision by reiterating the value of such modifications in maintaining her health, and helping her to visualize the lifestyle changes. At this point, the patient has already gathered and considered facts about the complications of diabetes and the necessary behavioral modifications. To move her to the next stage of the behavior change process, encouragement and advice on possible immediate lifestyle changes probably would be considered more relevant than would further basic educational information. The Transtheoretical Model focuses attention on the immediate stage of behavior of the patient, providing suggestions for stage-specific recommendations relevant to the patient at that point in time. Recommendations appropriate for and meaningful to the patient during the precontemplation stage (information on the disease and risk factors) may not be meaningful for the patient during the preparation stage (encouragement and reinforcement on decision to change behavior). Movement forward between stages can be considered a "success" despite lack of evidence of full behavior change by the patient.

Use of the Transtheoretical Model at the Population Level

A population-level study [17] of 50 patients with a hemoglobin A_{1c} of at least 9.0% were offered a choice of educational interventions such as a comprehensive diabetes management program, small-group education at a diabetes education center or at a primary care clinic, individual education at a diabetes education center or at a primary care clinic, telephone-based or fax-based education, or specific diabetes help through a health care hotline. Prior to beginning the educational intervention, the stage of change of each patient was measured. Following the intervention, individuals at the preparation and action stage had a mean reduction of over 2.0% hemoglobin A_{1c} within a 3-month period, whereas those in the precontemplation or contemplation stage had a mean reduction of only 0.61% hemoglobin A_{1c} in 3 months. The investigators [17] concluded that a simple tool that could gauge a patient's stage of change "could be used to target patients for educational programs more effectively and to design diabetes interventions more acceptable for both the patient and health care provider." The authors [17] proposed tailoring messages in the educational interventions to appeal to patients in the different stages of change.

EXAMPLE OF A COMBINATION OF MODELS

Models can be combined in entirety or in pieces to understand preventive, treatment, and maintenance behavior. For example, initial questions for a patient may be derived from the Transtheoretical Model as a basis to understanding the individual's current willingness to change behavior. Once his or her stage of change is established, one may inquire more specifically about psychosocial and environmental factors—described in the Health Belief Model—that may influence the current stage of change.

Use of a Combination of Models at the Individual Level

A 56-year-old woman, during a clinic visit, states that she has never had a mammogram. She says that she has no family history of cancer and does not feel that she needs a mammogram. She also has heard that the test is uncomfortable, and because she has no family history, she does not want to subject herself to the pain. However, she is considering having a mammogram within the next 6 months because her friend was diagnosed recently with breast cancer. According to the Health Belief Model, the patient does not perceive herself to be susceptible to the disease, and the fear of pain during the mammogram is a barrier in seeking the screen.

According to the Transtheoretical Model, the patient is considered to be in the contemplation stage of change. She is in the process of committing to a behavior change—to have a mammogram to screen for breast cancer within the next 6 months. Within the context of the Theory of Reasoned Action and Theory of Planned Behavior Models, the patient is increasing her behavioral intention through an evaluation of behavioral outcomes due to the news that her friend has been diagnosed with breast cancer (Fig. 3) [18].

The Theory of Reasoned Action Model and the Theory of Planned Behavior differ from the other models in their emphasis on motivational factors influencing behavior change. The Theory of Reasoned Action Model includes attitudinal and social normative factors influencing the behavior. The Theory of Planned Behavior includes all components of the Theory of Reasoned Action with the addition of perceived control of the behavior. Therefore, the new information about her friend's breast cancer provided the patient with a normative belief that mammograms are

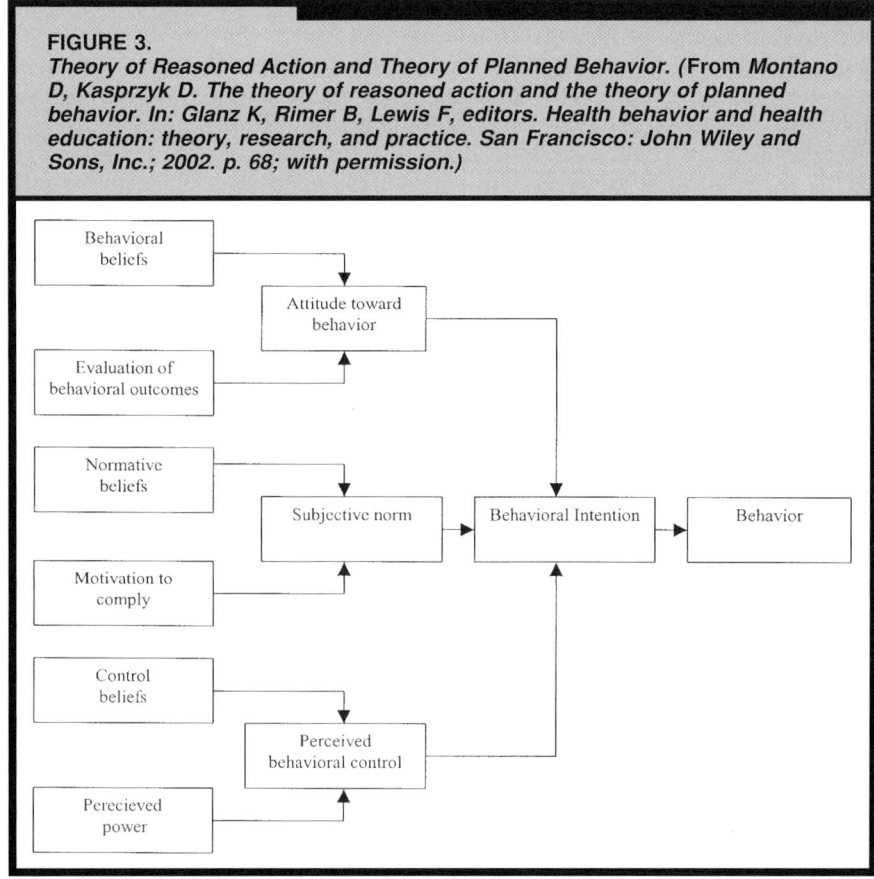

FIGURE 3.
Theory of Reasoned Action and Theory of Planned Behavior. (From Montano D, Kasprzyk D. The theory of reasoned action and the theory of planned behavior. In: Glanz K, Rimer B, Lewis F, editors. Health behavior and health education: theory, research, and practice. San Francisco: John Wiley and Sons, Inc.; 2002. p. 68; with permission.)

acceptable, improving her attitude toward the behavior, and motivation to adhere to the recommendation.

Strategies to address both the psychosocial and stage of change models would include provision of further information on the patient's actual susceptibility, information on the process of mammography to lessen fears of pain, and encouragement in the patient's decision to seek a mammogram in the next 6 months.

Use of a Combination Models at the Population Level

Champion et al [19] compared several interventions designed to increase mammography screening in nonadherent older women. Women between 50 and 85 years of age who had not had a mammogram within the past 15 months and had no history of breast cancer were recruited from health maintenance organizations and general medicine clinics. The women's stage of behavior change was assessed and an intervention was selected based on the stage. Depending on the stage of mammography adoption (Transtheoretical Model) and individual beliefs (Health Belief Model), women were provided either telephone or in-person counseling by a nurse or a mammography recommendation letter from their primary care physician.

In-person counseling in conjunction with the physician letter was significantly associated with increased adherence in women in the precontemplative stage, with an odds ratio of 5.19 compared with women with no intervention. The only significant predictor of mammography adherence in the contemplation group was membership in a health maintenance organization, although the odds ratios for all interventions, except the physician letter alone, were over 1.35 compared with the nonintervention group. The study [19] found that personal counseling had the greatest overall impact on adherence, but phone counseling also increased adherence by twofold and the nontailored physician letter had an additive effect for both the in-person and telephone counseling.

SELECTION OF AN APPROPRIATE MODEL

Selection of an appropriate model depends on factors such as the type of information sought by the physician and patient and preferred and available interventions. Many models are designed to address behavior change in the global sense, including preventive and screening behavior, treatment behavior, and maintenance behavior. However, models may vary in the degree to which they focus on psychosocial factors, social factors, environmental factors, stage of change, and type of associated interventions. Physician preference also may influence the selection of models. If one is interested in specific aspects of patient behavior—such as the relationship between perceived susceptibility to disease and perceived threat of the disease, and the consequent likelihood of behavior change— then the Health Belief Model may be of most interest. Comprehensive reviews of models may be found in texts such as *Health Behavior and Health Education: Theory, Research, and Practice*, edited by Glanz, Rimer, and Lewis [12].

METHODS OF INTERVENTION BY THE FAMILY PHYSICIAN

Following identification of the various factors associated with behavior change, physicians can intervene thorough several channels of communication. Examples include in-person counseling, telephone reminders, tailored mailings of letters, postings of general health education materials in a clinic or on a Web site, small-group meetings such as support groups or classes, or even political action such as lobbying for state laws mandating breastfeeding rooms at the workplace and nonsmoking public areas.

RECOMMENDATIONS FOR INCLUSION OF HEALTH BEHAVIOR MODELS

Focus groups with regional primary care physician opinion leaders in western New York found that the primary care physicians' perceived role in daily practice is as a "one-stop-shop" physician, but with an immediate focus on diagnoses and treatment [20]. The authors [20] discovered that

> Physicians believed implementing patient behavior change required changing the patient's mindset, including leading patients to accept more personal responsibility for their wellness. Yet, significant barriers to behavior change were related to physicians themselves. [Physicians] acknowledged their lack of training, knowledge, and skill in behavior change process and recommendation conveyance.

One respondent from the study stated, "So there's a lot that we have to learn that we weren't adequately trained for in terms of those difficult ways of motivating patients to stop smoking, lose weight, all that kind of thing" [20].

Health behavior models provide a simple tool for insight into the illness experience of a patient, identification of possible nonclinical factors affecting behavior change, and suggested interventions for patients and physicians. Mechanic [6] advises medical educators "to introduce aspiring doctors to a broader conception of practice and to give them more supervised experience in dealing with psychosocial factors and issues affecting function and the quality of life." Health behavior models are a useful tool for such instruction in medical schools, residencies, and continuing medical education. These models function at an individual level for understanding factors affecting patient illness and behavior, and at a population level for understanding a patient population and identifying population-level intervention strategies. Use of health behavioral models also can enable physicians and practices to evaluate outcomes such as patient function and satisfaction, in addition to traditional measures of morbidity and mortality.

In the words of Arthur Kleinman [7]

> It is clinically useful to learn how to interpret the patient's and family's perspective on illness. Indeed, the interpretation of narratives of illness experience, I will argue, is a core task in the work of doctoring, although the skill has atrophied in biomedical training. . .illness has meaning; and to understand how it obtains meaning is to understand something fundamental about illness, about care, and perhaps about life generally. Moreover, an interpretation of illness is something that patients, families, and practitioners need to undertake together.

Key Points

- Family physicians are the first points of contact in the health care system for many individuals and have a great responsibility to identify factors associated with the health status of a patient.
- Health behavior models provide a framework to identify various components—including demographic, psychosocial, and environmental factors—that may affect a patient's behavior.
- By selecting an appropriate health behavior model or a combination of models, family physicians can identify both specific factors affecting behavior change and the stage of change of a patient.
- Understanding psychosocial and environmental factors affecting behavior change, as well as stage of change, enables a family physician to select an appropriate preventive action or intervention for a patient.
- Interventions can include individual-level, group-level, community-level, or structural-level components depending on the needs of a patient and available resources.

References

[1] American Academy of Family Physicians. Policy and advocacy. Available at: http://www.aafp.org/x6809.xml. Accessed June 1, 2003.
[2] American Academy of Family Physicians. 2003 facts about family practice. Available at: http://www.aafp.org/x530.xml. Accessed June 1, 2003.
[3] Minino A, Smith B. Deaths: preliminary data for 2000. National Vital Statistics Reports 2001;49(12):1–40.
[4] Saelens BE, Sallis JF, Wilfley DE, et al. Behavioral weight control for overweight adolescents initiated in primary care. Obes Res 2002;10(1):22–32.
[5] Lyznicki JM, Young DC, Riggs JA, Davis RM. Obesity: assessment and management in primary care. Am Fam Physician 2001;63(11):2185–96.
[6] Mechanic D. Sociological dimensions of illness behavior. Soc Sci Med 1995;41(9):1207–16.
[7] Kleinman A. The illness narratives: suffering, health, and the human condition. New York: Basic Books, Inc; 1988.
[8] Dea RA. The integration of primary care and behavioral healthcare in northern California Kaiser-Permanente. Psychiatr Q 2000;71(1):17–29.
[9] Strosahl K, Robinson P, Heinrich RL, et al. New dimensions in behavioral health/primary care integration. HMO Practice 1994;8(4):176–9.
[10] Druss B, Mechanic D. Should visit length be used as a quality indicator in primary care? Lancet 2003;361(9364):1148.
[11] Flocke SA, Orzano AJ, Selinger HA, et al. Does managed care restrictiveness affect the perceived quality of primary care? A report from ASPN. Ambulatory Sentinel Practice Network. J Fam Pract 1999;48(10):762–8.
[12] Glanz K, Rimer BK, Lewis FM, editors. Health behavior and health education: theory, research, and practice. San Francisco: John Wiley and Sons, Inc., 2002.
[13] Patterson R. Changing patient behavior: improving outcomes in health and disease management. Chicago: Jossey-Bass; 2001.
[14] Janz N, Champion V, Strecher V. The health belief model. In: Glanz K, Rimer B, Lewis F, editors. Health behavior and health education: theory, research and practice. San Francisco: John Wiley and Sons, Inc., 2002. p. 52.
[15] McDonald-Miszczak L, Wister AV, Gutman GM. Self-care among older adults: an analysis of the objective and subjective illness contexts. J Aging Health 2001;13(1):120–45.

[16] Prochaska JO, Redding CA, Evers KE. The transtheoretical model and stages and change. In: Glanz K, Rimer B, Lewis F, editors. Health behavior and health education: theory, research, and practice. San Francisco: John Wiley and Sons, Inc.; 2002. p. 107.
[17] Peterson KA, Hughes M. Readiness to change and clinical success in a diabetes educational program. J Am Board Fam Pract 2002;15(4):266–71.
[18] Montano D, Kasprzyk D. The theory of reasoned action and the theory of planned behavior. In: Glanz K, Rimer B, Lewis F, editors. Health behavior and health education: theory, research, and practice. San Francisco: John Wiley and Sons, Inc.; 2002. p. 68.
[19] Champion V, Maraj M, Hui S, et al. Comparison of tailored interventions to increase mammography screening in nonadherent older women. Prev Med 2003;36(2):150–8.
[20] Mirand AL, Beehler GP, Kuo CL, Mahoney MC. Explaining the de-prioritization of primary prevention: physicians' perceptions of their role in the delivery of primary care. BMC Public Health 2003;3(1):15.

Address reprint requests to

Rebecca A. Malouin, PhD, MPH
Division of Epidemiology Services
Michigan Department of Community Health
3423 N. Martin Luther King Jr. Boulevard
P.O. Box 30195
Lansing, MI 48909

e-mail: malouinr@michigan.gov

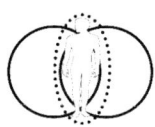

PROFESSIONAL AND PRACTICE MANAGEMENT SKILLS 1522–5720/03 $15.00 + .00

MEASURING AND IMPROVING CUSTOMER SATISFACTION

Devorah E. Rich, PhD

Modern medicine has come a long way. Major surgeries—such as coronary artery bypass graft or knee replacements—that once necessitated multiweek hospital stays, now allow patients to leave within days of the operation. What has not changed at all, however, is the need for excellent communication. Procedures that may be commonplace and routine to physicians, nurses, and other support staff can be a complete mystery to patients and their families. When a family member visits a hospital and a nurse comes in to check a monitor, providing the patient and family with information is critical to promoting their confidence and enhancing the quality of their experience.

Professionally, I measure customer satisfaction among customers of the University of Michigan Health System (UMHS). Recently, I had the opportunity to experience medical care from the other side, as a family member of a loved one. Sitting at my mother's bedside, I found that nurses fell into two broad categories: those that care about the patient or their family member and those that do not. A friend summed up hospital staff similarly as "those who like people and those who don't." Following an episode in which nursing care was particularly disappointing, a nurse manager inquired about my mother's "current nurse." I described her as "ok," adding that she was rather cold and a poor communicator. In her defense, the nurse manager stated that this nurse was very "competent." I viewed this as irrelevant. No patient or family member comes to a hospital and expects the nursing staff to be incompetent. That would be akin to buying a car and feeling grateful that it has four wheels. Pleasing the patient or family member extends beyond technical competence. The key to having a successful medical practice or hospital is communicating with patients and looking for ways to delight them.

From the University of Michigan Health System, University of Michigan Medical School, Ann Arbor, Michigan

Enhancing customer satisfaction demands constant effort. Soliciting customer feedback—whether through focus groups, one-on-one conversations, or formal surveys that can provide statistically quantifiable feedback—is paramount when designing systems that meet customer needs. These systems are critical to providing quality care. Staff members vary in the extent to which they will strive naturally to please patients. With system regulation and expectations, ambiguity is eliminated and standards of customer satisfaction can be monitored. Without systems, one is left to the nature of each individual. Many organizations are lucky enough to have staff that are caring, kind, and genuinely seem to like people; however, to avoid the concern of inconsistencies based on the personalities of the staff, it is paramount to have built-in systems and explicitly defined expectations for delivering customer service. This article discusses ways to obtain customer feedback so that you know what your patients and customers want and can continue to delight them. Obtaining customer feedback begins with identifying your customers. In health care, customers typically include patients, staff, referring physicians, employers, and insurance companies.

Patient satisfaction surveys commonly are used to provide measures of the quality of care from a patient perspective. Formal measurement of patient satisfaction is recorded in the literature as early as 1968 [1], but began to proliferate in the 1980s and 1990s. A review of the PubMed internet database [2] found a total of 22,242 international journal articles relevant to patient satisfaction worldwide. Some of the diverse topics pertaining to patient satisfaction included its connection with clinical outcomes [3,4], the impact of gender on patient satisfaction [5], and whether patient satisfaction is influenced by physician dress [6].

Patient satisfaction has evolved from an instrument used internally by organizations to a measurement that is shared with the public. The US government is in the process of developing a national survey tool to be used by all hospitals. Pilot testing of this survey instrument began in May 2003 in the states of New York, Maryland, and Arizona. The Centers for Medicare and Medicaid Services is initiating efforts to make comparative performance information on hospitals publicly available. The aim of this endeavor is twofold: to help consumers make more informed choices when selecting a hospital for care and to create incentives for hospitals to improve the care they provide.

METHODOLOGY

The UMHS has been measuring customer satisfaction systematically since 1985. Over the past 2 decades, the methodology has evolved so that the process of obtaining customer feedback is incorporated into quality-improvement initiatives. The measurement system that the UMHS has developed provides patient feedback to small and large offices, inpatient units, ambulatory care surgical sites, and ancillary services. This article outlines the UMHS's process of defining customer groups; developing measurement instruments; analyzing results; applying results to operations; and, finally, refining the measurement instruments as needed to assess both patient satisfaction and the impact of process changes on patient satisfaction.

The first step in measuring customer satisfaction is to define the research objectives. Customer research is an expensive endeavor and without clear objectives, useful results are difficult to obtain. Defining objectives can be accomplished through brainstorming around a particular topic. It often is useful to have an outside party lead this discussion, because an external perspective can be helpful in clearly articulating objectives. In addition, an outside party will probe continually to clearly articulate what needs to be asked. This will increase the likelihood of obtaining useful information. This process can be compared with a physician asking a patient, "What hurts?" The physician then needs to probe further to understand the real problem.

Similarly, persistent probing is a necessary step toward identifying research objectives. For example, "I want to know how to improve the care I give to my adolescent patients" is a vague objective. With probing, clarity can be improved, resulting in an objective like this one: "I am developing a program to target the health needs of adolescent patients. I would like teenagers to identify health issues that are important to them, and to identify what it takes for them to be comfortable disclosing sensitive and private information that can be very pertinent to treating their needs."

Typical customer groups include patients and their families, employees, referring physicians, and third-party payers (ie, insurance companies and employers). Depending on the type of practice, students and institutions that place the students also could be included in the customer group. Once the target audience has been identified, the next step is to identify the appropriate data-gathering method. Several options are available, but the most typical methods used in health care include focus groups and surveys. Focus groups typically are conducted to gain a deeper understanding of a specific subject or for an evaluation of something that is best done face to face. Surveys are conducted when quantifiable results that can be extrapolated to an entire population are desired. Surveys can be general and address all aspects of care or more focused if improvement initiatives are under way and it is important to measure their efficacy.

Focus Groups

Focus groups are best described as "informal but structured discussions." Focus groups typically involve 8 to 12 participants and are run by a trained focus group moderator. They are used for gaining in-depth understanding of how particular groups feel about specific issues or for testing promotional campaigns. Focus groups are informative and exciting to observe because they allow the client to obtain the customer's view, in his or her own words. They provide excellent and in-depth insight into the subject being studied. Focus groups can work for any size practice. The determining criteria in deciding if this is an appropriate methodology is an understanding of the type of information the practice wants to solicit from existing or potential patients. Focus groups should be used only when a practice is seeking in-depth patient feedback on a specific subject (eg, an advertising campaign or growth opportunities in a new market), or in-depth feedback from patients on how to enhance the medical services provided. For example, a medical practice might elect to use focus groups if they are contemplating expanding the practice to include more executive health screening services or perhaps want to target sports medicine. Focus groups can help to identify what potential patients and possibly companies are looking for when they contract with practices for these services. In both cases, the practice would want multiple focus groups, to discuss the needs of both patients and employers.

Table 1 outlines the steps involved in conducting focus groups. Several key factors are involved in successful focus groups, including clear objectives for information requested, an experienced moderator, and an adequate number of participants. As noted above, an external person often is very helpful in identifying objectives. In the initial meeting with the moderator or consultant, it is critical to identify the research objectives and then determine the number of focus groups to conduct.

TABLE 1.
Focus Group Process

Step	Factor/objective
Step 1	Meet with moderator to define focus group objectives
	Identify the required number of focus groups and criteria for including participants
	Determine focus group logistics
	• Location
	• Time
	• Refreshments
	• Amount of compensation
	• Method of recording (videotape, audiotape, court reporter)
Step 2	Reconvene with moderator to review:
	• Moderator's guide
	• Recruitment screener
	• Recruitment letter
Step 3	Recruit participants
	• Call list of participants
	• Mail confirmation letter
	• Call the day before to confirm participation
	• Arrange for payment to participants (cash, gift certificate)
Step 4	Focus group sessions
	• Observe through one-way mirror or video camera
	• Moderator takes a break half way through to see whether observers have any questions
Step 5	Transcription of focus group tapes
Step 6	Report and recommendations prepared and presented to client

Homogeneity among the participants is vital when conducting focus groups, to ensure the comfort of all participants. The definition of homogeneity will vary. For example, if a hospital is developing a new prenatal program and wants feedback from pregnant women, it is critical that there is at least two groups: one of first-time mothers and the other of pregnant women who previously have given birth. Otherwise, the experienced mothers can easily dominate the focus group, making it extremely difficult to obtain feedback from the first-time mothers. Likewise, in conducting focus groups among employees, it is critical to run different groups of staff, managers, and physicians. The number of focus groups conducted depends on the issue being examined and how many different constituency groups you need to hear from.

Focus group costs vary, but usually range from $2,000 to $5,000 per group, depending on the type of groups. Factors influencing the costs include (1) the focus group room (professional rooms with one-way mirrors are more expensive than are conference rooms), (2) difficulty of recruitment (physicians are the most difficult group to recruit), (3) the amount of money necessary to compensate participants (staff usually are not an additional cost during work time, but physicians tend to be the most expensive group to recruit, upward of $200 per person), and (4) the type of recording being conducted. Focus groups can be videotaped, audiotaped, or recorded by a court reporter, who sits in the room and records all comments. Recording costs vary, with the court reporter mode being the most expensive and the audiotaping mode the least expensive. Additional costs include transcribing the tapes (necessary for audiotaping and videotaping) and providing food for participants and observers. With audiotaping and videotaping, it is important that multiple microphones (connected into one recorder) be set on the table so that the person transcribing the tape can clearly hear what has been said. Focus groups are difficult to transcribe because in the excitement of the conversation, it is not uncommon to have multiple people talk simultaneously. Multiple microphones also allow the transcriber to hear soft-spoken participants.

Before conducting a focus group, the focus group moderator meets with the client and discusses the research goals. The moderator then drafts a moderator's guide, which is a series of questions that the moderator will ask. The moderator's guide is critical to the success of the final results, ensuring that the same questions are asked in each group. Because focus groups are, by nature, guided but free-flowing conversations, it is important that the client observe the focus groups to make sure that the moderator probes appropriately, particularly as unexpected issues arise.

Surveys

Although focus groups provide in-depth qualitative information, the results cannot be generalized to the population at large. In contrast, surveys provide quantifiable information that can be trended over time and, if the sample is selected correctly, generalized to a larger population than the group being surveyed. The ability to trend information over time or to measure the impact of a process change requires formal surveys that are standardized. These surveys ask the same questions and use uniform methodology from period to period or before and after a specific intervention.

Survey questions are divided into two main types: closed ended and open ended. Closed-ended questions use a scale, typically a two-point scale (yes/no) or a multiple-point scale. A Likert scale has at least five points, with a neutral point in the middle (eg, "strongly agree" to "strongly disagree," with a point in the middle labeled "neither agree nor disagree").

In developing surveys, the greater the number of points on the scale, the more "stable" the survey is over time. This implies that changes seen over time are likely to result from real changes in participant attitudes as opposed to measurement error. When developing survey questions, it is important that each question be clear, only measure one point, and be written at a language level that is appropriate for the audience. Pretesting the survey is necessary to ensure that the questions measure what you intend them to measure. An advantage of working with a national or regional vendor is that they often can provide surveys that are used by a number of organizations, and benchmark data can be obtained to see where a particular organization stands relative to the benchmarks.

Open-ended questions invite comments. Typical examples include: "If you could change one thing about the care you received today, what would it be?" These questions are useful in that they provide many ideas from your survey group that you may not have thought of. Unfortunately, the results cannot really be trended, and the researcher cannot extrapolate the ideas to the population at large. However, with enough of the same comments, the survey may be modified later to measure the extent to which the population at large is concerned about an issue raised through individual comments.

Distribution Methods

Many methods for obtaining customer feedback are available. It is important to use the methodology that will provide the maximum amount of feedback for the minimum price, and in a manner that does not antagonize customers. Table 2 outlines the various survey methods and their pros and cons.

The typical survey methods are mail, telephone, point of service, and Internet. The Internet is the least expensive method of surveying and works well for employees (assuming the culture supports e-mail and Web activities). It essentially is free, and there are no data entry requirements.

The point-of-service method is the second least expensive survey method. With this method, the survey is distributed and collected personally at the time of the service encounter. This is feasible if staff are available to distribute and collect the surveys. The University of Michigan uses this method among ambulatory clinic patients. These

TABLE 2.
Survey Data Collection Methodology Comparisons

Data Collection Methodology	Cost	Distribution Requirements	Response Rate	Ideal Audience
Mail	$1.50/ survey	Easy	30%–40%	Patients with a procedures
Telephone	$50–$70/ survey	Easy	80% of households reached	Referring physicians, general public, employers, insurance companies
Point of service	$1.25/ survey	Staff intensive	65%	Patients with clinic visit
Internet	$2.25/ survey	Easy	30%–50%	Employees, students

surveys are distributed twice a year for a 1-week period, with every clinic patient receiving a survey. In total, approximately 60% of the patients respond. The high volume (usually 14,000 surveys are returned in 1 week) allows for analysis of the data at the specialty and subspecialty level, and physician-specific level. However, because this data collection method is time consuming for the staff, it is limited to a 1-week period twice a year. This methodology is recommended only for surveys controlled by the office. If a practice is working with an external vendor, the best methodology is mail or telephone, because when you work with an external vendor, one of the advantages is receiving data contrasting your practice with others. It is difficult to have consistent distribution methods between different offices for the point-of-service methodology. Therefore, a more traditional (but expensive) method such as mail or telephone is preferred.

The method of regular mail is effective when the population is interested in participating and willing to return the survey. It is expensive because of the two-way mailing costs (sending and providing postage-paid return envelopes); the response rate usually is around 30% to 40%. Telephone surveys, the final method, can be quite expensive depending on who the target audience is. However, this is frequently the only way of reaching this audience. Phone surveys are necessary for referring physicians, employers, insurance companies, and for community-at-large surveys (eg, public awareness).

The Appendix provides a simple survey to measure patient satisfaction with an office visit. The survey, subdivided into four parts, measures the key elements of a patient's visit. The first section addresses access. The second and lengthiest part of the survey addresses the patient–physician interaction. This section is the longest because the only reason the patient makes an office visit is for this interaction. Hence, measuring how well physicians perform relative to the patient–physician interaction is critical.

The next section concerns cleanliness of the facilities. Patients may not know if the medical care is appropriate. However, if the examination room or restrooms are dirty, this is a red flag to patients that the medical care may be substandard. Although there may be no actual correlation between cleanliness and the quality of medical care, when a patient has no other means of judging the medical care, cleanliness is the first litmus test the office must pass to assure patients that they will receive quality medical care. The final section summarizes the patients overall assessment of their appointment. By asking questions about overall satisfaction with the care received and willingness to recommend, the practice receives a good sense of how well it is doing. The willingness to recommend question is paramount and always should be included, because the threshold for recommending is higher than the threshold for returning. That is, inertia, may keep dissatisfied patients returning to your practice, but they are much less likely to recommend the practice to others. After all, it is their name that is on the line.

Data Analyses

Upon completion of the survey, the results can be analyzed in different ways, varying in complexity. The ability to analyze survey results and turn the data into useful information depends on the method of data collection. Ideally, each survey should be linked to the patient who completed it. This linking will facilitate more complex analyses—such as connecting patient satisfaction with medical outcomes—allowing for precise targeting of interventions.

The simplest analyses to perform include the basic statistics of frequency distributions and means. Frequency distributions are useful because they allow the investigator/researcher to clearly see how people responded to each question. When conducting mean summaries, the UMHS has moved toward presenting all means as a 100-point mean index rather than a straight mean. When a question is posed on a 5-point scale, the 100-point mean index converts the 5-point scale to a 100-point scale ranging from 0 to 100, with a 25-point spread for each of the items on the 5-point scale. Hence, the conversion is 1 = 0, 2 = 25, 3 = 50, 4 = 75, and 5 = 100. When viewed from the language of the scale, this means that strongly disagree becomes 0 and strongly agree becomes 100. With this method, it is much easier for people reviewing the information to understand the meaning of a 77 as opposed to a 3.67. The other advantage is that it easily summarizes all of the responses into one number, so that when they are tracked over time, is easier to understand the direction of change. At the University of Michigan, researchers focus the trending of data on the 100-point mean index, but always present the frequency distributions so that managers can see the distribution spread.

Often these simple statistical measures are sufficient. Many managers can use this overall information to develop specific improvement strategies for their overall population. If appropriate, however, the second level of analysis is to compare survey results between time periods. This is done most typically through a chi-square test or an analysis of variance (ANOVA) test. The chi-square tests the hypothesis that the row and column variables are independent, without indicating strength or direction of the relationship. This test compares changes in frequency distributions over time. The Pearson chi-square is used most commonly to detect statistically significant changes over time. Although it will indicate whether there is a significant change, the original frequency table is needed to determine the direction of change.

Another test that is used frequently is the ANOVA. The ANOVA tests the null hypothesis that several group means are equal in the population by comparing the sample variance estimated between the group means to that estimated within the group means. When evaluating these results, researchers focus on the P value as a means of deciding whether to accept or reject the null hypothesis. The P value refers to the observed probability that a statistical result will occur if the null hypothesis is true. If the observed significance level is small (ie, unlikely) enough—usually less than 0.05 or 0.01—then the null hypothesis is rejected.

The chi-square test and the ANOVA test simply provide information with regard to whether there has been a change in any of the measured items over time. They also can be used within a given time period to detect differences between subpopulations. For example, these tests might look for differences in how men versus women or younger versus older people perceive different aspects of the care received.

More sophisticated statistical analyses are used to help prioritize improvements. This can be done through multiple regression models, in which a series of independent variables are measured in relationship to their impact on the dependent variable. Typical dependent variables may include willingness to recommend the clinic to others, overall satisfaction with the care received, and overall satisfaction with the supervisor. These regression models can be run for each appropriate subgroup, such as medical department, gender, or race. For example, among oncology patients, a key factor in satisfaction with the care may be pain management, whereas among primary care patients, the key factor may be communication. Whatever the key factors, identifying them and sharing this information with administrators and clinicians is critical for improving service delivery.

The UMHS uses a partial least square regression model to identify improvement priorities for patients and employees. This model, which begins by using factor analysis to cluster like items together, quantifies the impact of each survey question on overall patient loyalty. A partial least square regression model, although extremely useful in prioritizing strategies and distinguishing differences by subgroup, is a proprietary model owned by only two companies and is extremely costly. The model quantifies the expected impact of each factor and each item within the factor on improving patient loyalty. This is quite helpful, because it can be used to clearly set priorities and to identify how much money to allocate to specific improvement endeavors, based on their expected impact. For example, an organization may assume that scheduling problems are the greatest source of patient dissatisfaction. However, the model may reveal another factor to be more significant. Hence, the model can determine the most efficient allocation of resources. This model, summarized in Fig. 1, resonates well with physicians because it is extremely quantitative.

In reviewing the model in Fig. 1, the goal is to increase patient loyalty (defined as willingness to recommend and willingness to return). The "drivers" in box B and C impact the loyalty box. The greater the impact score (underlined), the greater the impact. Hence, it is clear that Quality of Care has a greater impact on patient loyalty than does Visit Comparison (ie, how this health facility compares with others the patient has been to). To the left of the drivers are the subdrivers, which impact the drivers. Provider Satisfaction measures the patient satisfaction with their physician or nurse practitioner. It is clear that this has the greatest impact on the Quality of Care (3.4 as compared with Scheduling, which only has an impact of 0.2) Hence, it is easy to see where one would target resources for improvement. Improving the scheduling system would only be worthwhile if it could be done easily and inexpensively.

In addition, by running models for each department, unit, or job category, the model can identify key drivers for each different constituency. Table 3 identifies key drivers of employee satisfaction by employee job category. When developing improvement plans, it is critical to realize that "one size does not fit all." Tailoring the improvement strategies to the specific groups involved increases the likelihood of success.

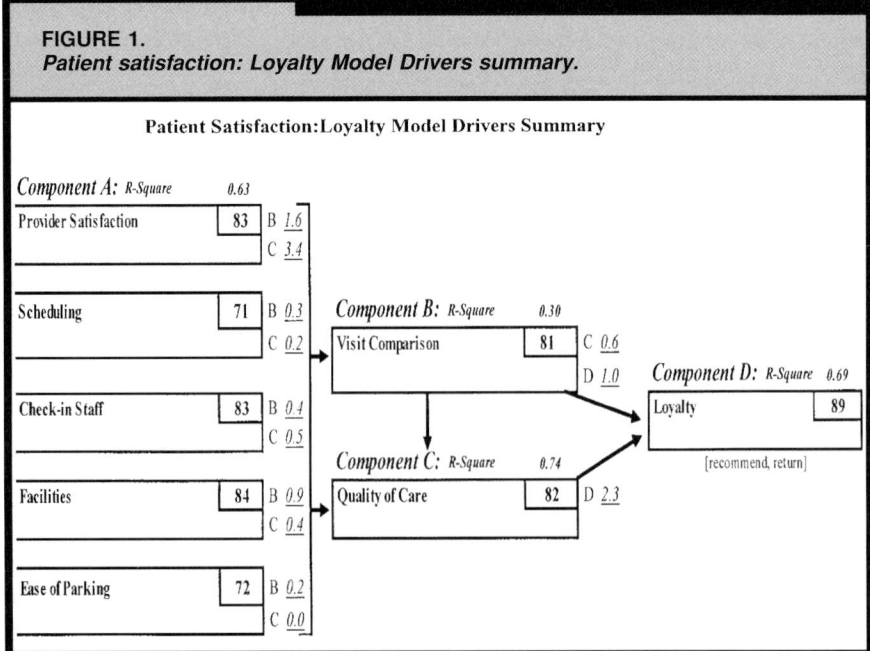

FIGURE 1.
Patient satisfaction: Loyalty Model Drivers summary.

	Allied Health	Professional and Administrative	Nurse	Office	Service Maintenance
TABLE 3. *Priority Differences by Job*					
Relations with supervisor	X	X		X	X
Recognition	X	X			X
Relations with coworkers		X	X	X	

This model is used at the UMHS for both patient and employee satisfaction. Table 3 suggests that with a staff composed of nurses and office staff, improving relationships with coworkers would be an important priority. Given limited resources, issues that cross multiple job categories would take precedence. If the staff were composed of Professional/Administrative and Office employees, appropriate areas of concern would be either relationships with supervisors or relationships with coworkers. Recognition, on the other hand, is less of a priority for the office staff.

At the University of Michigan, the partial least square regression model is run every few years, because the results are unlikely to change and identifying the key drivers and subdrivers of change is most important.

Distributing Survey Results

Research results, whether surveys or focus groups, should be shared at all levels at which they impact staff. Survey reports should be prepared at the level at which they impact employees, so that appropriate improvement actions can be taken. For example, reports at the subspecialty area or by unit in the inpatient arena will be much more useful to staff at that level who want to make change. Likewise, physician-specific survey results have a powerful impact. People are much more motivated to initiate change when they feel that the results address them personally. It is too easy to disregard general results as being about others.

At the University of Michigan, one department that started with a low patient satisfaction rate became the star department within a 1-year time frame. This occurred because the survey results were shared with all of the staff, a Process Improvement Team used the regression model results to identify and focus on priorities for improvement, and the department chair shared the results with each physician and made public each physician's satisfaction ratings. Although this may seem unduly harsh, the chairman felt that physicians are very competitive people and would be more likely to improve if their results were posted for all to see.

Using Survey Results to Implement Change

Sometimes it is helpful to link patient satisfaction data to medical outcomes so that interventions can be targeted to specific populations. This can be achieved if there is a link between the survey and a patient. Numbering the surveys, keeping a record of which patient received which survey number, or stamping a patient's identification number directly on the survey are ways in which this can be facilitated. Patients should be told that although the surveys are not anonymous, all the information they provide is completely confidential. Sometimes, in reviewing patient comments, a caring physician or staff member may request the name of a patient who expressed a particular grievance, to follow-up and resolve any lingering patient concerns. Unless the patient has explicitly provided his or her name and requested that someone contact them, this is illegal and the researcher is not permitted to disclose this information.

With the introduction of the Health Insurance Portability and Accountability Act (HIPAA) privacy laws, it is critical that patients be informed that the information being collected through the survey is being used only for quality improvement initiatives. It is advisable to have the patients sign, as part of the HIPAA consent form information, a statement agreeing to participate in surveys that may be linked to their name for the exclusive purposes of quality improvement initiatives only.

Successfully implementing organizational process changes based on feedback received from customer surveys has two components. First, a project champion (an enthusiastic leader who will direct the project) instills confidence in the staff and has the ability to garner any necessary resources required to implement change. Second, the process should be co-championed by an administrator and a physician or nurse, depending on the situation. Including an administrator is very important, because he or she often is able to maneuver the changes within the system.

In the following two examples, the UMHS successfully made operational changes using the combination of patient satisfaction data and patient demographic information. The first example took place in a multidisciplinary ambulatory breast care clinic. A survey was distributed to evaluate patient perceptions of multidisciplinary medical care. All patients seen in this setting were surveyed over a 3-month period. The surveys were numbered and results were tied to a clinical database that included the indicators of age, diagnosis, first or repeat visit, referral source, second opinion, and family history of breast cancer. Results indicated a significant difference in satisfaction based on whether patients were diagnosed as benign or malignant. Interestingly, the patients diagnosed as benign were much less satisfied. Further investigation showed that their dissatisfaction was caused by excessive wait times, both to receive an appointment and to be seen at the time of the appointment. According to an analysis of differences in wait time among these two populations, patients suspected of having a malignant tumor had an average wait time of 14.6 days for their scheduled appointment, compared with 31.8 days for patients suspected of having a benign tumor. To rectify this problem, a separate adjunct clinic was set up with nurse practitioners who were able to screen patients suspected of having a benign tumor. This shortened the wait time considerably. Here, the quality improvement initiative was implemented as a direct result of the knowledge gained by combining patient satisfaction with clinical outcomes.

The second example, focusing on the inpatient perspective, concerned obstetric patients. An analysis of patient satisfaction compared women who delivered through cesarean sections with women who delivered vaginally. The inpatient satisfaction survey was precoded to connect patient satisfaction with Diagnostic Related Group (DRG) information to facilitate the analyses. Chi-square tests were run on the frequency distributions between the groups. Results indicated that women with cesarean sections were significantly less satisfied than were women who delivered vaginally. The team charged with developing improvement plans further hypothesized that there would be a statistically significant difference between women who had planned and unplanned cesarean sections. To conduct this analysis, the medical records of all cesarean section women in the survey were examined. The cesarean section women then were categorized by whether the procedure was planned or unplanned. Results indicated that women with unplanned cesarean sections were significantly less satisfied than were women with planned cesarean sections.

To address these findings, a clinical nurse specialist was assigned to check on women with unplanned cesarean sections three to five times before their discharge. The clinical nurse specialist would visit each woman and make sure she felt comfortable about the cesarean section. For women with unplanned cesarean sections, the emotions and disappointments were intense, and the University of Michigan found that simply giving them this time increased their satisfaction.

In addition, further analysis revealed a significant need for "Just-in-Time" learning despite all the prenatal education that women receive. Upon delivering their babies, women were overwhelmed by a host of questions that they had not considered previously. This resulted in the development of a discharge-planning course, which provided an opportunity for new mothers to come with their babies and any adult family members they desired (spouse, grandparent, or friend) to ask the questions that arise once the baby is a reality.

Keys to Successfully Implementing Change

Sharing survey results with staff is the first step to successfully implementing change. This is true especially when the results are disappointing. Improvement can take place even when departments do nothing more than share results. Sharing results indicates openness to staff input and a willingness to be candid about where things currently stand.

The next key to success is interest on the part of the leadership. The leadership should assemble a multidisciplinary improvement team to represent the various groups that interact together to provide quality service, with physician and administrator leadership. This dual leadership is important; physicians greatly influence the environment of the office or unit, and administrators can garner necessary resources to make changes. Other staff should be selected for participation based on their interest and excitement to be a part of the improvement process. Although staff often are identified by a particular job that they do at work, their talents generally extend beyond the limits of their job description. Participation in an improvement task force can reveal many of these external qualities not typically used in the workplace, and watching them flourish can be an exciting process. It is important to bear in mind, however, that any organizational reorganization initially will have an adverse impact on employee satisfaction. Hence, when reorganizing processes and people, it is extremely important to pay attention to potential adverse impacts and work to minimize these impacts (on both staff and patients). Table 4 summarizes the keys to success.

Impact of Satisfied Employees

Satisfied customers are vital to the success of an organization, and satisfied customers begin with satisfied employees. According to a study performed at the UMHS, employee satisfaction and patient satisfaction are significantly correlated. Not surprisingly, this study also revealed a significant correlation between high employee satisfaction and low employee turnover. Departments that reported high employee satisfaction had half as much turnover as did those departments with low employee satisfaction (14% versus 7%, respectively). In addition, the average cost of employee turnover per employee was found to be between $6,800 and $20,000, depending on the training level of the employee. Clearly, it is quite important to focus on customer satisfaction among all groups, including employees, patients, insurance companies, and referring physicians.

It is interesting to note the paramount importance of good communication, whether with employees, patients, families, or others. When people

TABLE 4.
Keys to Successful Implementation of Change

Factors Positively Impacting Change	Factors Negatively Impacting Change
Communicating results to staff	Unwillingness to share customer feedback with staff
Involving staff in improvement efforts	Departmental reorganization
Providing leadership opportunities for staff	Departmental staffing changes
Creating a multidisciplinary improvement team with physician and administrative leadership	

feel that they are receiving information, they are better able to cope with difficult or disappointing situations. The research studies conducted at the UMHS reveal direct links between employee satisfaction and low turnover, and between employee satisfaction and patient satisfaction. Understanding the processes that impact patient and employee satisfaction allows management to set up a process so that employees know what is expected of them. The result will be an organization with more consistent staff, reflecting the values and goals of the organization, rather than the personality and daily ups and downs of each employee.

Monitoring customer satisfaction takes constant effort. This article outlines the steps involved in different measurement processes. Successful customer research programs not only measure the attitudes and experiences of the various customer groups, but then take that information and use it to make improvements. The final steps in the improvement process are communicating these actions back to the customer and measuring for improvement. When communicating with customers, be open and explicit. Let them know, that "they talked, you listened, and here is what's new." Customers will not only be more forgiving of problems they encounter when they feel people are listening, but they will want to partner with you. This type of scenario will lead to a win–win situation in which happy staff lead to happy patients, and happy patients invigorate the staff. The end result will be a more successful and satisfying medical practice for all connected with it.

Key Points

- Customer satisfaction is paramount to an organization's ability to survive and to thrive in very competitive times. Customers are defined as both internal (employees) and external (patients, employers, referring physicians, and so forth).
- There is a strong positive correlation between employee satisfaction and patient satisfaction. In addition, satisfied staff improve an organization's bottom line by having lower employee turnover.
- Periodic and consistent measurement of customer satisfaction permits organizations to understand the needs of each customer group, and to make process changes that allow organizations to meet and exceed the expectations of their customers.

References

[1] Korsch BM, Gozzi EK, Francis V. Gaps in doctor–patient communication. Pediatrics 1968;42(5):855–71.
[2] National center for biotechnology information. Pub Med database. Available at: http://www.ncbi.nlm.nih.gov/entrez/query.fcgi?term=PatientSatisfaction. Accessed May 5, 2003.

[3] August DA, Ehrlich D, Carpenter LC. Patient evaluation of care within a multidisciplinary breast care center. Quality Management in Health Care 1993;3(3):1–15.
[4] Bonnema J, van Wersch A, van Geel AN, Pruyn JF, Schmitz, Paul MA, et al. Medical and psychosocial effects of early discharge after breast cancer: randomised trial. Br Med J 1998;25:316(7140).
[5] Weisman CS, Rich DE, Rogers J, Crawford KG, Grayson CE, Henderson JT, et al. Gender and patient satisfaction with primary care: tuning in to the women in quality measurement. Journal of Women's Health and Gender-Based Medicine 2000;9(6):657–65.
[6] Li SF, Haber M, Birnbaum A. Patient satisfaction and physician dress in the emergency department. Academic Emergency Medicine 2003;10(5):550.

Address reprint requests to
Deborah E. Rich, PhD
University of Michigan Health System
6319 Med Science 1
University of Michigan Medical School
Ann Arbor, MI 48109-0642

e-mail: debrich@umich.edu

APPENDIX

Sample Office Survey

Your opinions matter. Please answer the following questions about the care you received today.

Calling the office check-in	Poor	Fair	Good	Very Good	Excellent
1. Length of time between making an appointment and the day of your visit	☐	☐	☐	☐	☐
2. Helpfulness of check-in staff scheduled appointment	☐	☐	☐	☐	☐
Length of time at office/clinic from until seeing the doctor	☐	☐	☐	☐	☐
Appointment: Doctor 3. Personal interest shown in you and your medial problems	☐	☐	☐	☐	☐

4. Doctor's ability to answer questions in a way that you could understand ☐ ☐ ☐ ☐ ☐

5. Thoroughness of the examination/ treatment ☐ ☐ ☐ ☐ ☐

6. Explanations of medical procedures and tests ☐ ☐ ☐ ☐ ☐

7. Amount of time you spent with the doctor during your visit ☐ ☐ ☐ ☐ ☐

8. Overall satisfaction with the nursing care ☐ ☐ ☐ ☐ ☐

Facilities

9. Cleanliness of the restrooms ☐ ☐ ☐ ☐ ☐

10. Cleanliness of the examination room ☐ ☐ ☐ ☐ ☐

Overall rating

11. Overall, how would you rate the care you received at the office/clinic? ☐ ☐ ☐ ☐ ☐

	Definitely Not	Probably Not	Unsure	Probably Would	Definitely Would
12. Based on your most recent visit, would you recommend this office/clinic?	☐	☐	☐	☐	☐

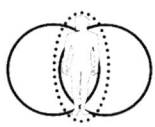

PROFESSIONAL AND PRACTICE MANAGEMENT SKILLS 1522–5720/03 $15.00 + .00

THE CHALLENGING PATIENT

Frederick W. Kron, MD, Michael D. Fetters, MD, MPH, MA,
and Edward B. Goldman, JD

"All nature is but art unknown to thee,
All change, direction which thou canst not see,
All discord, harmony not understood,
All partial evil, universal good"

—*An Essay on Man*, Alexander Pope

Every physician-patient encounter is challenging, a complex give -and take of many messages and metamessages. Family physicians generally are comfortable with the mainstream encounters that their personalities, training, and personal development allow them to understand and manage successfully. When encounters take on a more challenging flavor, however, the patient-care process and outcome can be stressful and unsuccessful for physician and patient alike. Family physicians therefore need to develop a broad repertoire of skills and a special depth of understanding to surmount the challenges that are an immutable feature of the patient-care landscape.

An estimated 15% of patients in physicians' practices are experienced as "frustrating" or "difficult" [1,2]. Consequently, a family physician who sees 20 to 30 patients a day on average will have approximately four to five challenging encounters a day—possibly more. Factor in the disproportionately large impact that these encounters often have on provider time and their potential emotional toll, and it is easy to develop a sense of the significance of dealing with challenging patients.

This article presents strategies to limit frustrations and increase effectiveness of care. Specific areas addressed include developing a sharpened understanding of challenging patient interactions, learning where problems are likely to occur, avoiding missteps that could exacerbate a challenging situation, and getting back on track should a faux pas occur.

From the Department of Family Medicine, University of Michigan Health System, Ann Arbor, Michigan (FWK and MDF); and the Office of the General Counsel, Health System Legal Office, University of Michigan, Ann Arbor, Michigan (EBG)

THE FAMILY MEDICINE PERSPECTIVE ON CHALLENGING PATIENT ENCOUNTERS: A COMPREHENSIVE VIEW

Doctors generally are trained to think in terms of a linear, biomedical model of disease [3,4], in which there is a logical sequence from symptoms to objective data to diagnosis, treatment, and cure. Physicians educated according to this model often feel frustrated when dealing with patients whose elusive problems are subtle markers for other less-obvious issues, or whose symptoms serve some purpose for them and are not generally amenable to cure.

What constitutes a challenge regarding certain patients is also conditioned by a host of other factors. Every specialty has its own unique point of view of so-called "problem patients": legal specialists caution physicians about refusing to care for troublesome patients whose behavior may expose their medical provider to liability, emergency medicine [5] factors prisoners and violent and homeless patients into the mix, and psychiatry focuses on personality disorders and borderline defenses [6]. In addition to being comprehensive in the age range of patients seen and in the breadth of illnesses treated, Family Medicine also promotes the integration of behavioral concepts and social issues into scientific, evidence-based patient care; that is, it embraces the biopsychosocial model. The family doctor's unique practice paradigm necessarily influences the types of challenges that may be encountered, and implies that he or she takes a more holistic, comprehensive approach to challenges when they arise. This means that the family physician needs to examine all of the component parts of challenging interactions—the contributions of the patient's physiology, psychology, and social situation to his or her overall health, as well as the physician's own contribution.

Patients usually are perceived to be challenging when encounters with them, or even just seeing their names on the daily schedule, provokes a negative reaction from the clinician. This can range from a sigh and a feeling of resignation to a gut-tightening feeling of outright disgust. In this sense, the challenging patient is defined by the clinician's reaction to that patient. But that reaction may well be conditioned by factors wholly unassociated with the patient per se. For example, physicians who place

---

Box 1. Examples of Provider Challenges

- Frustrating medical system
- Fatigue
- Illness
- Heavy schedule
- Interpersonal or financial problems
- Low value on the psychosocial aspects of patient care

low value on the psychosocial aspects of patient care experience more encounters as being difficult [1]. Female providers may experience more frustration when dealing with difficult patients than do their male counterparts [19]. In addition, physicians besieged by medical systems problems and clinicians whose psyches are battered down by sleep deprivation, interpersonal, financial, or their own health issues may be triggered more easily, and may consider patients as challenging whom they might not have otherwise, were they themselves not somehow challenged (Box 1).

How to Think About Challenging Patients

Creating a comprehensive list of all challenging patients, or even trying to categorize them definitively, is a daunting proposition. In his seminal 1978 article, Groves [7] developed four stereotypes of what he described as "hateful patients," which he labeled as dependant clingers, entitled demanders, manipulative help-rejecters, and self-destructive deniers. Since then, many different systems to characterize and classify patients who challenge health providers have been developed.

A useful way to approach the topic of challenging patient encounters is to think first about behaviors that are typically characterized as being challenging to medical providers (Box 2) [3,6,8], and then consider some of the psychologic and social issues that may bring about those behaviors (Box 3) [3].

Underlying all challenging behaviors, in one form or another, is neediness, which may also be coupled with some degree of dysfunctionality as to how the patient approaches getting his or her needs met. From the Family Medicine perspective, these patients are in biopsychosocial

---

Box 2. Examples of Challenging Patient Behaviors

- Multiple complaints involving multiple body systems
- Vague and shifting complaints
- Barrage of complaints
- Act on medical misinformation
- Dependent, clinging behavior
- Do not ever seem to get well
- Undue concern about minor symptoms
- High utilization of health care services
- Demanding, controlling, manipulative
- Overtly hostile
- Unrealistic expectations of cure
- Raises problems right at end of visit
- Noncompliant
- Rambling, unfocused, confusing
- Self-destructive
- Substance abuse

Box 3. Examples of Psychosocial Issues Underlying Challenging Patient Behaviors

- Feelings of guilt, worthlessness, incompetence, or shame
- Survivors of childhood abuse, sexual or other
- Victims of domestic violence
- Loneliness, social isolation
- Fear of abandonment
- Life stress (eg, job stress, divorce)
- Maladaptive defense mechanisms to cope with life stressors (Somatoform Disorder, Hypochondriasis)
- Mood disorders (anxiety, depression, panic, bipolar)
- Personality disorders (borderline, dependent, obsessive, paranoid)
- Involvement with tort law or workers' compensation system

---

disequilibrium [9]. They are merely trying to get their needs met and, ideally, to get back into balance.

TECHNIQUES TO DEAL WITH CHALLENGING PATIENTS: THE "ART" OF FAMILY MEDICINE

Rather than draft an excruciatingly detailed picture of every patient type and detail every conceivable intervention, we instead will paint a more impressionistic canvas of possible patient approaches. From this perspective, physicians may extract and use the techniques that they perceive are most appropriate, both from the standpoint of their styles and the protean predicaments they may encounter.

Avoid Passive or Active Patient Neglect

When dealing with challenging patients, do not just ignore them in the hope that they will simply go away. Taking this approach might actually exacerbate problem behavior; it also could result in actual patient harm.

Be Thorough

A patient may have maladaptive coping strategies, but he or she also may have a bona fide, organic disease. Thus, it is important to make sure that, at the outset, every patient gets the benefit of a comprehensive records review (including the records of previous providers), a careful physical examination, appropriate objective studies [10], and a complete psychosocial history. Look closely for the problems that sometimes may underlie challenging behaviors: shame or embarrassment about physical or sexual abuse; anxiety, depression, or bipolar disorder [1]; situational problems, such as social isolation, job stress, or marital strife; and any history of school failures, fights, and so forth that may suggest psychological problems or personality disorders.

Self-Awareness

Physicians traditionally have fixed the blame for challenging encounters on the "problem patient." As we've indicated, it is more realistic to view a challenging encounter as resulting from a blend of personalities and situational factors. Most often, the problem is not in any one individual factor; it is somewhere in the mix.

If you find yourself triggered by a challenging encounter, do not just look at the patient as the source of the problem: look inward. The third law of the *House of God* states: "At a cardiac arrest, the first procedure is to take your own pulse" [11]. Take stock of yourself. Be introspective. Recognizing and working out personal issues will help to increase emotional reserves when dealing with the daily challenges of medical practice. Participation in Balint groups [12,13] may be useful in this regard. Seeking support from peers or mental health professionals also may be helpful.

Be aware of when stress levels rise. Controlling negative emotions is a prerequisite to the ethical treatment of patients. Remain calm, confident, and in control, and avoid acting out of anger or frustration.

When a patient encounter is growing tense, it may be useful to take a break, get some space, and reassess the situation. Leave the room, or reschedule the visit if necessary, to regain the energy and clarity necessary for managing a challenging situation.

Avoid Labeling

There is no evidence to suggest that physicians can promote change by persuading patients to admit to a diagnostic label. On the contrary, accusing patients of being "in denial," "resistant," or "dysfunctional" is far more likely to increase their resistance and encourage argumentation than to instill trust and motivation for change [14].

There often is a temptation to apply negative labels to challenging patients. You've probably heard frustrated physicians venting about "crocks" or "gomers." First, consider that these derogatory epithets are no less offensive than are racial epithets, which one would never expect to hear in a physician's office [5]. Moreover, when you voice negative characterizations, you tend to strengthen them subconsciously. In the lingo of social psychology, "As I speak, I learn what I believe" [14]. Instead, we suggest that physicians opt for the ethical high ground, and make it a rigid discipline to always show respect for their patient's underlying humanity.

Maintain Healthy Boundaries

When treating a patient, be compassionate, but do not become so passionate that you risk emotional exhaustion by enmeshing yourself in the patient's problems. (That is, do not make the patient's problems your problems.) Maintaining sufficient emotional separation will help you to objectively consider your patient's issues, and find medically acceptable approaches consistent with the patient's values. Also, set reasonable limits on appointment times and communicate these clearly to your patient. People sometimes may see appropriate boundary setting as a rejection, so be prepared to deal with this in a firm yet compassionate manner.

Practice Patience and Capitalize on Continuity

When beginning treatment with a new patient, be aware that getting a clear sense of the patient's actual problem may take several appointments. Do not expect an epiphany on the first visit. Also recognize that patients with seemingly irresolvable problems often benefit simply from the ongoing, caring relationship with their physician. The "therapeutic containment" offered by the provider visit—that is, the opportunity to feel safe and secure in a caring environment—may be all that the patient really is looking for.

Schedule Frequent, Brief Visits and Set Goals for Each Visit That Are Limited and Mutual

Setting regular appointments at 2- or 3-week intervals may ease dependent patients' anxieties. Routine contact also makes it less likely that patients will present with new or persistent symptoms [8]. To keep appointments focused and effective, have patients write down and prioritize their health concerns beforehand. This encourages patient self-efficacy and, by crossing items off the list, serves to illustrate that progress is being made. Restrict the number of problems to be covered during a visit to a manageable number, and actively involve the patient in the decision about which problems to cover on a given day. This will help to cultivate a sense of physician-patient partnership.

Partnerships, the physician-patient variety among them, generally will not accomplish much if the partners have different agendas. Many conflicts arise from a lack of shared goals. When clear goals are established, agreement about the means to achieve them is reached much more easily. The patient-care corollary is that to avoid conflict and work together productively, you should ascertain that you and your patients share mutual goals for care.

Finally, set limited goals for care. Do not promise big improvements, and do not expect them, either. Keep objectives small and manageable. Celebrate successes.

Activate Support Services As Appropriate

Patient education, whether Internet based (eg, the website of the American Academy of Family Practice, www.aafp.org), or by means of more traditional classes and written handouts, may help the patient who has health concerns. Social work, psychology, psychiatry, and other disciplines including alternative medicine providers, can also be useful allies for patients struggling through difficult life circumstances.

As pointed out earlier, situational stress often sends people into the downward spiral of psychosocial disequilibrium and can lead to mal-adaptive coping strategies such as projection or somatization [9]. Helping patients to cope successfully with stress through the use of stress-management techniques can help to restore psychologic equilibrium, and may contribute to improved mental and physical health [15]. Short-term psychologic stress counseling or stress clinics can be very helpful in this respect.

Although a psychiatric referral usually is not necessary, in select circumstances, clinching a psychiatric diagnosis may help to delineate a specific approach that might make your care more effective.

Consider Using Motivational Interviewing Techniques

Motivational Interviewing (MI) [14] presents providers with a critically important set of skills that they can use to help their patients recognize and change problem behaviors. It builds on the client-centered philosophy of Carl Rogers, who sought to provide a safe and supportive atmosphere in which patients could explore their experiences openly and reach resolutions to their own problems. MI then goes a step further, finding practical and strategic ways to facilitate the patient's expression of self-motivational statements, thereby encouraging the patient, rather than the doctor, to present arguments for change.

Even though it was devised in the setting of addiction counseling, the principles and techniques of MI can be applied to a wide array of problems. The five general principles of MI are presented in Box 4 [14].

Although a full discussion of MI is beyond the scope of this article, it is hoped that the list of general principles will provoke thoughtfulness and,

---

Box 4. Principles of MI

- Employ empathy
- Develop discrepancy
- Avoid argumentation
- Roll with (patient's) resistance
- Support self-efficacy

hopefully, entice the reader into learning more about this useful change stratagem.

Demonstrate Physician Behaviors That Build Trust

Your manner should be comforting and caring. Ask the patient questions, both to learn more about him or her and to test your understanding of his or her meaning. Answer the patient's questions as thoroughly as possible. When doing an examination or a procedure, always explain what you are doing. Finally, demonstrate competency [16].

WHEN ALL ELSE FAILS: HOW TO END THE PHYSICIAN-PATIENT RELATIONSHIP

Despite your best efforts, you cannot remediate effectively every challenging situation. It is essential to be genuine and to recognize when your abilities have been exceeded. It also may be that the challenging individual provokes issues with nursing, support staff, or even with other patients that are of such magnitude that the only viable option is to respectfully terminate that patient from your practice.

Although a patient can end the physician-patient relationship at any time and for any reason, a physician who wants to dismiss a challenging patient must be far more deliberate. Physicians cannot end a relationship with a patient for legally impermissible reasons, such as age, race, sex, religion, or medical conditions (eg, AIDS) that are entitled to protection under the American's with Disability Act. Furthermore, state law may provide specific requirements that must be met. The following general guidelines, although not state specific [17], nonetheless should help to keep providers safely within the realm of both ethical and medico-legal correctness.

Behavioral Contracts

If a patient is uncooperative, you may want to make a behavioral contract with him or her. Behavioral contracts may help to encourage patient compliance; also, should legal action arise from the termination of a physician-patient relationship, the courts are more inclined to look with favor on providers who have "gone the extra mile" to assist challenging patients by offering them behavioral contracts. This is illustrated by the case of *Payton v Weaver* [18], in which the court allowed a dialysis center to discontinue caring for a noncompliant dialysis patient who failed to follow a behavioral contract.

Document Diligently

Behavioral contracts should be documented in the patient's medical record and signed by the patient. If the patient breaches the contract, this also should be documented clearly. Indeed, all discussions (including telephone discussions) and all the facts that pertain to a problem behavior should be recorded carefully in the patient's medical record.

How to Notify the Patient

Once you have decided to end a relationship with a patient, you should communicate this to the patient in writing. Ideally, letters should be sent by certified mail, return receipt requested. If the patient refuses to claim the letter, try handing it to the patient during an office visit; if that is not possible, then the letter should be sent to the patient via first-class mail. The letter should explain that you will no longer provide care for the patient. However, it should not say why this action is being taken; any explanation could allow the patient to disagree and even to claim defamation of character.

No Sudden Stops

You must tell the patient that the relationship is being ended with sufficient time for the patient to arrange for other medical care. If there is a need for ongoing care, this should be spelled out clearly in your letter (eg, "Because of your diabetes, you need to have annual eye exams..."). You also must offer to be available for a specified period of time during which the patient can establish care with another provider. Although 30 days usually is adequate, the precise time frame will depend on the circumstances of each case.

No Specific Provider Recommendations

You should suggest various places, such as the state or county medical society, where the patient can get lists of local physicians from whom he or she may obtain care. There are two reasons why you should avoid making a specific provider recommendation: (1) the new provider may encounter the same difficulties and may blame you for "dumping" an unwanted patient; and (2) if the new provider is not satisfactory, the patient may allege that you made an inappropriate referral, resulting in a claim of injury.

Offer to Transfer Medical Records

It is important that patient records be transferred so as to ensure continuity of care.

The sample letter in Box 5 illustrates this principle and the other principles described above with regard to terminating with a patient.

Box 5. Sample Termination Letter

Dear [Patient's Name],

I have been pleased to be your physician in the past, but I must inform you that I am withdrawing from providing further professional care for you.

Because your condition requires ongoing medical care [give details as necessary], you should make arrangements to find another physician as soon as possible. If you require a referral, you may wish to contact the [State of Country] Medical Society Physician Referral Service at [phone number].

If you wish, I will continue to be available to treat you while you are transferring your care to another physician. However, this period will not exceed 30 days from the date of this letter. This will provide you with ample time to select a new physician.

Upon receipt of your written authorization, I will provide your new physician with a copy of your records and information regarding the services I have provided.

Sincerely,

Signed: Dated:

Key Points

- A family physician who sees 20 to 30 patients a day on average will have approximately four to five challenging encounters a day.
- Family physicians need to examine all of the component parts of challenging interactions—the contributions of the patient's physiology, psychology, and social situation to his or her overall health and their own contribution.
- A number of strategies are available to family physicians to help make caring for challenging patients more rewarding.
- In instances in which the physician-patient relationship cannot be remedied, it may be necessary to terminate it.
- A series of procedures can be followed to keep providers who terminate the physician-patient relationship safely within the boundaries of ethical and legal propriety.

References

[1] Jackson JL, Kroenke K. Difficult patient encounters in the ambulatory clinic: clinical predictors and outcomes. Arch Intern Med 1999;159(10):1069–75.
[2] Hahn SR, Kroenke K, Spitzer RL, et al. The difficult patient: prevalence, psychopathology, and functional impairment. J Gen Intern Med 1996;11:1–8.
[3] Gillette RD. "Problem patients": a fresh look at an old vexation. Fam Pract Manage 2000;7(7):57–62.
[4] Rakel RE, editor. Practicing biopsychosocial medicine. In: Textbook of family practice. Philadelphia: WB Saunders; 1995. p. 55–60.

[5] Simon JR, Dwyer J, Goldfrank LR. Ethical issues in emergency medicine: the difficult patient. Emerg Med Clin North Am 1999;17(2):354–71.
[6] Noble J. Classification. In: Textbook of primary care medicine. 3rd edition. Mosby; 2001. p. 459–62.
[7] Groves JE. Taking care of the hateful patient. N Engl J Med 1978;298:883–7.
[8] Haas LJ, Sanyer ON, White GL. Caring for the frustrating patient. Clin Rev 2001; 11(10):75–8.
[9] Rakel RE, editor. Psychosocial influences on health. In: Textbook of family practice. Philadelphia: WB Saunders; 1995. p. 46–54.
[10] Gillette RD. Caring for frequent-visit patients. Fam Pract Manage 2003;10(5):57–62.
[11] Shem S. The house of God. New York: Dell; 1979.
[12] Balint M. The doctor, his patient, and the illness. 2nd edition. London: Pitman Books, Ltd.; 1964.
[13] Balint E, et al. The doctor, the patient, and the group. Balint revisited. London: Tavistock/Routledge; 1993.
[14] Miller WR, Rollnick S. Motivational interviewing: preparing people for change. New York: Guilford Press; 2002.
[15] Vogel ME, Romano SE. Behavioral medicine. Prim Care 1999;26(2):385–400.
[16] Thom DH. Stanford Trust Study Physicians. Physician behaviors that predict patient trust. J Fam Pract 2001;50:323–8.
[17] University of Michigan Policies. Medical abandonment: ending the physician-patient relationship without legal consequences. Unpublished data.
[18] *Payton v Weaver*, 131 Cal. App. 3d 38 (1982).
[19] Levinson W, Stiles WB, Inui TS, Engle R. Physician frustration in communicating with patients. MedCo 1993;31:285–95.

Address reprint requests to

Frederick W. Kron, MD
Department of Family Medicine
University of Michigan Health System
1500 E. Medical Center Drive
Room L2003, Box 0239
Ann Arbor, MI 48109-0239

e-mail: mfetters@umich.edu

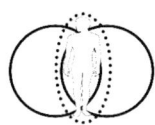

PROFESSIONAL AND PRACTICE MANAGEMENT SKILLS 1522–5720/03 $15.00 + .00

MEDICAL–LEGAL ISSUES: THE PATIENT RELATIONSHIP AND RISK MANAGEMENT

Rebecca W. West, JD

The law interfaces with many aspects of medicine, from business-related issues of billing to the legal structure of the practice, and from malpractice to Federal regulations such as the Health Insurance Portability and Accountability Act (HIPAA) and the Emergency Medical Treatment and Active Labor Act. Whether you are just starting your practice or have been in practice for some time, these issues will have a significant impact on your practice. Although this article cannot focus on all these issues, those presently in the forefront of the news—such as quality of care, malpractice issues, and new regulations such as the HIPAA's privacy provisions—are discussed. This article endeavors to provide the family practitioner with a good understanding of the basic issues, focusing on risk management strategies for the private family practice clinic.

The term malpractice refers to professional misconduct, defined as unreasonable lack of skill or fidelity in carrying out professional or fiduciary duties. Although the word fiduciary most often is associated with financial responsibilities, it actually refers to the duty of care that a person is held to when entrusted with something that belongs to another person. In the medical context, fiduciary refers to the duty that a physician has to a patient who has entrusted his or her medical care to a physician. The purpose of the medical malpractice lawsuit is to afford recovery for injuries suffered when physicians fail to exercise ordinary and reasonable care in the diagnosis and treatment of patient [1]. Lawsuits for patient care also may be brought on other grounds, including breach of confidentiality (in some states, this is considered a part of medical malpractice claims, whereas in other states. it is considered a separate cause of action),

From the Piedmont Liability Trust, Charlottesville, Virginia; and the University of Virginia School of Medicine, Charlottesville, Virginia

Portions of this article are drawn from material previously produced by Ms. West for the Piedmont Liability Trust, Charlottesville, Virginia. The material is reprinted with permission of the Piedmont Liability Trust.

product liability, contract liability (failure to meet a promise or guarantee), or vicarious liability (liability for the acts of another under your supervision or control).

Negligence is the most common of the theories used to sue a physician. To succeed on a theory of negligence, a plaintiff must establish by a preponderance of the evidence (greater than 50% likelihood) that the physician has a duty to the patient, that the physician breached the duty, and that the breach was a proximate cause of resulting injuries.

Usually, there is no dispute as to whether a physician–patient relationship exists. When a patient accepts professional services rendered by a physician, the physician–patient relationship is established. No explicit agreement is required. In general, the relationship does not exist until the physician sees the patient. One of the issues this article explores in more detail is what this duty to treat means and how the relationship, once created, may be terminated appropriately. Other issues also may arise. For instance, an on-call physician who does not respond when called may well be liable for injury resulting to a patient who was in need of the physician's services. Moreover, if medical advice is given over the telephone, even if the patient is not seen, a patient relationship most likely has been created. Conversely, a patient relationship most likely has not been created if the physician simply responds to a consult request by a physician colleague and never sees the patient or his or her medical records and delivers no care or treatment.

Proving that there is a breach of the applicable standard of care is a two-step process. First, the standard of care must be defined and then evidence must be introduced to show that the physician's care fell below the applicable standard of care. Competing plaintiff's and defense experts will assert what a reasonable physician under similar circumstances should have done for the patient. Authoritative texts or professional policies or standards also may be used to establish the applicable standard of care. Ultimately, a jury will determine what evidence is more credible and whether a breach of the standard of care has been proved.

If a breach of the standard of care is found, the plaintiff also must prove that it was more likely than not that this breach caused the plaintiff's injuries. Legal causation is divided into two categories: cause-in-fact and proximate cause. Cause-in-fact merely means that injury would not have occurred "but for" the physician's negligence. Proximate cause means that the physician's negligence was a "substantial factor" in bringing about the patient's injuries. Expert testimony again is used to prove this element of negligence.

The final element of proof in the plaintiff's case is damages. Damages may include physician, financial, or emotional injury to the patient or his or her immediate family. The purpose of the damage award is to compensate the plaintiff for injury with payment of a monetary award. Punitive damages may be awarded if the facts show the negligence to be gross or if malice, fraud, or wanton or intentional conduct is established. Punitive damages are not related directly to, or necessarily proportionate to, the injury suffered by the patient, but are intended to punish the defendant. In some states, damages have been capped in medical malpractice actions. Such caps may be on noneconomic damages (pain and suffering); on punitive damages; or, in a few instances, be a cap of the total damages of any type that may be awarded in a medical malpractice case. Such damage caps have been the subject of much discussion in the medical community and in the legislation, particularly in times of a medical malpractice insurance crisis.

If a case proceeds to trial, a jury will decide whether the plaintiff has established all the elements of the case and what the damages will be.

HISTORIC CONTEXT

Before the 1950s, medical malpractice lawsuits were relatively rare. Between 1950 and 1960, they increased at a rate of 2% to 5% annually. In the 1970s, the medical malpractice insurance marketplace was very tight financially. Insurance companies pulled out of a number of markets, leaving physicians unable to purchase insurance. Some state medical associations formed their own professional liability companies. By the end of the decade, the medical malpractice insurance market had improved.

Then in the 1980s, premiums skyrocketed. State medical associations pushed for tort reform—both legislative and regulatory. These tort reform efforts included caps on noneconomic damages, requirements for certificates of merit to be filed with a medical malpractice lawsuit, limits on contingency fees, reductions in statutes of limitations, and standards for expert witnesses. Success in passing tort reform varied greatly from state to state. By the 1990s, the medical malpractice insurance market had stabilized again. Access to coverage was not a problem, competition among the insurance carriers flourished and kept premiums under control, and the number of lawsuits being filed remained relatively stable during this period. Strong investment returns and a good economy also helped to keep premiums stable.

However, by 2001, the medical malpractice environment was turning toward another crisis. A fragile stock market decreased investment returns for insurance companies, the number of lawsuits began increasing somewhat, and jury verdicts increased significantly. All of these factors led to significant increases in medical malpractice insurance premiums. Insurers also began leaving the marketplace again. St. Paul Insurance was the largest underwriter of physician coverage historically, but suddenly found this line of business to be insufficiently profitable; therefore, St. Paul withdrew from the medical malpractice insurance market. A number of other insurance companies felt financial stress. Notably, Reciprocal of America was placed in receivership. Some states were losing physicians, and a significant number of states experienced large increases in premiums. A large actuarial company, Tillinghast, projected tort costs to increase two times as fast as did the economy in general. PriceWaterhouseCoopers reported that 7% of new health care costs would be associated with medical malpractice litigation [2].

The Department of Health and Human Services (HHS) reported that the average award in medical malpractice cases rose 76% from 1996 to 1999. HHS reported the median award in 1999 to be $800,000, which was a 6.7% increase from the prior year. Moreover, between 1999 and 2000, the median awards were said to have increased 43%. Again, tort reform took center stage with a push for damage caps in state legislatures and at the federal level being at the center of discussions. This time, however, the discussions also included a focus on quality of care issues and a drive to reduce medical errors [3].

THE QUALITY INITIATIVE

The Institute of Medicine (IOM) was established in 1970 by the National Academy of Sciences. It acts under the auspices of the Congressional Charter given to the National Academy of Sciences and is an advisor to the federal government to identify issues of medical care, research, and education. The IOM has taken the lead in the quality of care initiative. The initial report of the IOM stated that annually between 44,000 and 98,000 preventable hospital deaths were due to medical errors [4]. It also stated that annually between 3% and 38% of hospitalized patients were affected by iatrogenic injury. On average, it was reported that 7% of hospitalized patients suffered adverse drug events. This same report also stated that more people die from medical errors each year than from breast cancer, AIDS, or motor vehicles accidents [4].

It is clear that the public is paying attention to these reports. A Kaiser Foundation Study in 2000 found that 51% of the American public is following media coverage on medical errors closely; the federal government is watching these reports closely as well. The Center for Medicare Services (formally the Department of Health and Human Resources) has stated that quality is one of its foci as well and is a basis for fraud and abuse under the federal False Claims Act. Industry also has picked up the quality initiative, as best exemplified by the Leap Frog Group, which is a voluntary group of major US companies that have come together for the purpose of improving health care and with a goal of controlling the cost of health care as a by-product. The IOM put forward 10 guidelines to care, which are as follows [4]:

Continuous healing relationship
Customized care for patients
Patient as the source of control of care
Information regarding care flows freely
Decision-making regarding care is evidence-based
Safety is a system property
Transparency of medical errors
Needs anticipated
Waste continually decreased
Cooperation among providers and patient is a priority

The present quality-improvement movement will be driven by the following:

Information technology (focus first on on-line medication ordering systems)

Payment mechanisms (eg, Leap Frog companies [Fortune 500 businesses that have voluntarily come together for the purpose of trying to improve the quality of health care] will reimburse only for care that meets certain standards)

Clinical knowledge (movement toward evidence-based medicine)

Professional workforce

Legal/regulatory systems

Safe harbor for error reporting

Appropriate level of liability (eg, Enterprise liability)

Movement toward evidence-based medicine

As indicated, this focus on quality will appear in a variety of aspects of medicine and in a variety of legal mechanisms. One issue that remains open is the implications of more open discussions of errors and quality issues with a goal of improving health care systems when the legal system generally still holds the physician accountable in any professional liability civil case. Physicians will need to assess the benefit of openly discussing quality concerns with the risk posed by the use of such information to physician liability in claims.

ESTABLISHING A PATIENT RELATIONSHIP

Often questions arise as to when a physician–patient relationship is established; what the obligation to treat is once that relationship has been established; and, finally, under what circumstances the relationship can be severed. The answers to these questions are important because a physician can be held liable for abandonment if the physician–patient relationship is terminated inappropriately.

A Physician's Duty to Treat

As a general rule, a physician does not have a duty to treat anyone. However, once a physician first sees an individual and agrees to treat him or her, the physician–patient relationship is established and, with it, the physician's duty to treat the patient for his or her particular condition. The physician is obligated to provide treatment until this particular condition is resolved. Once this medical condition is resolved or treatment is complete, the physician–patient relationship may be severed. The physician need not do anything to notify the patient of the severance of the relationship, but instead may simply refuse to make further appointments should the patient request one.

Terminating the Relationship

If the physician wishes to terminate the physician–patient relationship before the completion of treatment, the physician may do so rightfully under most circumstances. The physician must notify the patient that he or she intends to break the physician–patient relationship and refer the patient to another physician. The patient must be given this notice with sufficient time to enlist the care of another physician without detriment to the patient. It is recommended that the physician notify the patient in writing, but if notification is given in person, the discussion should be documented.

A physician generally is justified in making arrangements for a qualified substitute to render care to his or her patients when he or she is unavailable, provided that the physician notifies the patient in advance and the patient agrees to the arrangement. When the physician is unavailable due to an unforeseen emergency, he or she generally will not be held liable for failure to attend to patients. Some patients believe they have a relationship with one particular attending in a large medical center and may allege abandonment when a resident or another attending sees them. However, most patients who go to medical centers for treatment reasonably should expect to be taken care of by multiple physicians.

Two exceptions to the right to terminate the physician–patient relationship are important to note. First, when the patient is pregnant and being treated for that condition, the physician generally does not have the right to terminate the relationship until the baby is born. Further, in the event of an emergency, the physician generally must provide treatment until the patient's condition stabilizes.

Abandonment

If a patient feels that the physician has terminated their relationship inappropriately, the patient may allege abandonment. Such an allegation generally is based on breach of contract. Because the action is based on a contract, the cap on damages in a malpractice tort action does not apply. Some courts have sustained such a cause of action as medical malpractice. To recover under either theory, the patient must prove that he or she was injured as a result of the abandonment. There are, however, circumstances in which the courts have refused to find abandonment. For example, if the physician was ill or physically unable to continue treatment, this may be seen as adequate reason not to have provided notice to the patient. A current example might be a physician in the military reserve who is called to active duty. Although the physician will be excused from the physician–patient relationship, if there is sufficient time, the law would require that notice and a referral to another physician be given to the patient. Similarly, a patient failing to cooperate with the prescribed treatment often is justification for termination of the relationship. Again, the patient should be given notice of the termination.

Courts generally will not look favorably on circumstances in which the physician–patient relationship was severed in mid-course because the patient did not pay for services. However, once treatment for the given condition is complete, the relationship may be terminated and treatment for future medical problems denied.

Good, clear communication with the patient is invaluable. The physician's actions will be viewed in light of what is reasonable in a given factual situation. Therefore, a physician should try to view his or her contemplated actions objectively before terminating a relationship with a patient.

In summary, a physician should not willfully terminate a relationship with a patient in the midst of treatment unless the situation falls clearly within one of the exceptions described above. After the treatment for the particular condition is completed, the relationship may be terminated safely. Finally, when termination is appropriate, it should be communicated in writing to avoid problems of proof.

CONFIDENTIALITY/PRIVACY

Patient privacy and confidentiality has become a nationally recognized right of patients with the Privacy Regulations effective April 14, 2003, that are a part of the HIPAA. These federal privacy regulations create a minimum national standard for privacy of protected health information (PHI). The regulations defer to state laws that may create a stricter standard than do the federal provisions, so that applicable laws still may vary from state to state based on each state's provisions. Although HIPAA does not give patients and their families a right to private lawsuit under its regulations, many states do recognize breach of confidentiality as a cause of action for which civil damages may be awarded.

Confidentiality has been considered basic to the physician–patient relationship, as is evident from the Hippocratic Oath [5]:

> Whatever, in connection with my professional service, or not in connection with it, I see or hear in life of men, which ought not to be spoken of abroad, I will not divulge, as reckoning that all such should be kept secret. While I continue to keep this Oath unviolated, may it be granted to me to enjoy life and the practice of the art, respected by all men, in all times, But should I trespass and violate this Oath, may the reverse be my lot.

The American Medical Association's modernized oath with regard to confidentiality is as follows: "That whatsoever you shall see or hear of the lives of men or women which is not fitting to be spoken, you will keep inviolably secret."

The HIPAA privacy regulations are intended to protect patient privacy and to allow patients a certain degree of control over their medical information. They are not intended to interfere with communications that are necessary in the course of sound medical practice.

HIPAA gives patients the right to

Receive a notice of privacy practices from their health care providers (and other Covered Entities)
Examine their own person health records
Request amendment of their records
Request limits on others' access to records
Receive communications by alternate means or at alternate locations
Know who has received their personal health information outside of their physician's practice for reasons other than treatment, payment, or health care operations

Under HIPAA, the health care provider must

Inform patients of their privacy practices (ie, provide written Notice of Privacy Practices)
Enact safeguards that protect privacy
Adopt privacy policies and procedures
Educate all staff about privacy practices
Appoint a privacy officer
Document privacy-related requests, complaints, and activities
Discipline employees who fail to comply

The HIPAA privacy regulations protect patient information in all forms, whether electronic data in computers, laptops, or personal digital assistants (PDAs); written documents; faxed documents; or oral communications. The HIPAA provides for civil or criminal penalties for noncompliance. These penalties can apply to organizations or individuals. Individuals or institutions may be

Fined up to $25,000 for multiple violations of the same standard in a calendar year.
Fined up to $250,000 or imprisoned for up to 10 years for knowing misuse of protected health information.

In addition, a practice is expected to discipline members of its workforce who violate the HIPAA privacy provisions, with such sanctions generally including suspension or even termination of employment.

The Notice of Privacy Practices (NOPP) is a written notice of how patient information is shared within your practice and with your business associates for treatment, payment, and business operations. Your clinic's NOPP should be provided to patients at the time they register with your clinic. Patients must be asked to sign an acknowledgment indicating that they received the NOPP.

So what is protected under HIPAA? PHI is medical information that can be identified as belonging to a particular individual—it is not just the patient's medical record! PHI is any combination of medical information and personal information such as:

Name
Medical record number

Social security number
Telephone number
Address
Birth date
Dates of admission, treatment, and discharge

However, it is important to remember that HIPAA allows health care providers to use and disclose PHI for the purposes of treatment, payment, and health care operations (TPO) without the patient's specific written authorization. Payment includes billing for services, submitting claims to insurance companies, and utilization reviews. Health care operations include activities related to quality assessment, training, underwriting, audits, compliance, business management, and certain general administrative tasks.

When the HIPAA allows the "use" of PHI, it allows PHI to be used by the organization for internal purposes only. Thus, with your practice, a doctor or other authorized person conducting a specific work function with PHI may "use" a patient's PHI without specific authorization by the patient. For example, a nurse may report laboratory test results to a physician, or a registration clerk may verify patient insurance information. Likewise, a quality improvement committee may discuss a patient's medical record. However, when PHI is shared, transferred, or revealed to someone outside of your practice, it is considered a "disclosure." If a practice uses or discloses PHI for purposes other than TPO, it will need written "authorization" from the patient, unless law states otherwise (eg, in response to court orders, subpoenas, or public health reporting). Authorization requires a written form that meets all HIPAA requirements and is signed by the patient. An example of a disclosure requiring patient authorization is a patient's request to release his or her medical records to a lawyer. It is worth noting that the HIPAA does allow disclosure of PHI to a patient's family and friends with regard to treatment or payment if:

The patient is present and has the opportunity to, but does not object.
The patient is not present or is incapacitated or incompetent, and disclosing the information is in the patient's best interests.

General information also may be disclosed for all patients, unless they expressly request that their information be restricted. For instance, a hospital may give out directory information, which is the name, location, and general condition (usually a one-word description such as fair) of the patient. A physician also may give patient treatment information to a patient's caregiver so that the caregiver can look after the patient at home. However, whenever PHI is used and disclosed, whole patient charts should not be turned over as a general response to a request for information on a patient. This concept is known as "minimum necessary" and provides that one should disclose only the minimum amount of PHI necessary for the requested purpose. This means that the registration staff in your clinic should have access only to patient information that they need to do their job. It also means that insurance companies should be given only information relevant to the charge they are reimbursing.

GOOD COMMUNICATION

Good communication and rapport with patients is very important for providing quality patient care and reducing risk exposures. Studies conducted to determine why patients sue providers suggest that it is the patient who perceives a poor relationship with their health care provider who is most likely to file a lawsuit [6].

Telephone Protocols

First Impressions

Telephone contact is likely to be the first interaction a patient has with your office. Whether dealing with a first-time patient or an established patient, the attitude projected by the person answering the telephone is crucial to creating and maintaining good patient rapport. Simple courtesies such as requesting permission to place a caller on hold with frequent checks made on holding lines assist in promoting positive perceptions.

Telephone Triage

It is advisable to develop written protocols for handling patient telephone calls. Office staff should know which calls to transfer immediately to the physician or nurse. Nonmedical personnel should never give medical advice. Some busy offices can handle medical questions through a precisely designed telephone screening and advice protocol.

Communication in the Office

The medical experience is, for many patients, alien and lonely and one that strips away a patient's perception of control. As such, the patient is particularly vulnerable in a medical environment. Although the reality of this situation may be more readily apparent in the hospital, the stressors that attend health problems are present in the outpatient setting as well. It is helpful to remember and to be sensitive to the patient's particular situation when communicating with the patient or family. Listening carefully is an indisputably valuable skill for any health care professional. Listening will allow for the collection of important information that might be unavailable otherwise, as well as provide the patient with the knowledge that they have been heard.

Communication Among Health Professionals

It is important to coordinate communication among those health professionals who are providing patient care. Breaks in communication are particularly easy when there is more than one service involved in caring for a patient. To the degree possible, it is helpful to coordinate medical terminology to avoid confusion or a perception by the patient that they have received conflicting information. Although there may be differences in opinion with regard to the best treatment options, these differences should be discussed outside of the hearing of patients or their families. Anxiety is amplified in a patient who overhears a discussion between health care professionals concerning their health care. Although patients may need to be presented with treatment options, a direct presentation of these options versus hearing these options debated are two entirely different experiences from the patient's perspective.

INFORMED CONSENT

Informed consent is a concept that originated in the courts in the United States in the 1950s. The basic common law concept of requiring a person to consent to touching by another person was expanded to recognize the fiduciary relationship between a physician and his or her patient and required the physician to provide the patient with certain information before the patient consented to the care or treatment by the physician.

As discussed, good patient communication and rapport is fundamental to a good physician–patient relationship. The informed consent process is the discussion that provides information that will allow a patient to determine within his or her own life experience, beliefs, and attitudes whether to opt for one treatment versus another or for no treatment. This process also is one of the key opportunities to establish a good rapport with the patient. Although patients may not remember the details of the consent discussion, they usually do remember whether their questions were answered and their concerns were addressed.

Elements of Consent

The basic elements of informed consent are that a physician must provide to the patient:

Their diagnosis
The nature and purposes of the proposed care or treatment
The risks and consequences of the proposed care or treatment
Alternative choices of care or treatment
The risks and consequences of no treatment

Informed consent may be expressed or implied. In most instances it must be given expressly by direct words, whether written or oral. Consent, on occasion, may be implied by reasonable inference based on the patient's actions. For example, a person who knowingly stands in line to receive a vaccination has implied consent to the vaccination. Most often the law does not direct whether informed consent must be in writing. When a statute does direct that written consent be obtained, the circumstances will vary from state to state (eg, some states require a patient's written consent to do HIV testing).

The most common exception to the requirement of a patient's informed consent is in an emergency. Emergency generally is interpreted relatively broadly to encompass instances in which delaying care to obtain informed consent likely will cause the patient to be at greater risk. This risk does not need to be a risk of death, but rather a greater risk in general to the patient's health.

General Rule

As a general rule, absent special circumstances, a patient has the right to refuse to authorize care or treatment, whether the refusal is grounded on doubt of success, concern for risks, lack of confidence in the health care providers, religious beliefs, or mere whim. Refusal of treatment on religious grounds has been recognized as a right of all individuals that is protected by the First Amendment of the Constitution. Under the Supreme Court's analysis, an adult of sound mind cannot be compelled to submit to medical treatment against his or her will unless the State can show a "compelling, overriding interest." When a child's care is involved, the State has been shown to have an interest in the welfare of the child, so although the parent's wishes most often will be honored, a court order overriding the parent's wishes may be sought based on the "best interests" of a child. In determining the best interests of a child, the court generally will look at the child's age, risks of treatment, benefits of treatment, likelihood of the benefit being achieved, and the likelihood of serious consequences if the treatment is withheld.

Minors

The general rule for minors is that consent of a minor to care or treatment is ineffective and consent must be obtained from the parent or person standing *in loco parentis* (in place of the parent as recognized by the law). However, if a minor is married legally, in active military service, or recognized by your state's law as emancipated legally, then the minor may consent to his or her own care. Difficulty arises with minors when they have been left in the temporary custody of another. In such instances, it is appropriate to treat the patient only if there is written consent of the parent permitting the person with temporary custody of the child to make health care decisions for that child or in the event of a medical emergency.

Another complication in the decision-making process with regard to minors is when they are held in the custody of social services. In such instances, state law will direct which agent of the department of social services may consent appropriately to the minor's care. If the minor has been placed with a foster family, the foster family generally is not the appropriate party to consent to care unless there is a court order directing that they make health care decisions. Moreover, when a minor has been removed to the custody of social services, a parent's right to make medical decisions for the minor has been removed, even if only temporarily and even if the child is allowed to visit the parent. Likewise, a noncustodial parent generally is not permitted to make medical decisions for a child, unless a court order or state law has provided otherwise. Rather, it generally is the custodial parent who makes medical decisions for the minor. It is worth noting, however, that a number of states do allow the noncustodial parent access to their child's records, even when they are not the decision maker.

Incapacitated Patients

When a patient is not competent to consent on his or her own behalf, "substituted" consent is obtained from the guardian, agent with a durable power of attorney (or health care power of attorney), or the next of kin. A patient will be considered incompetent if he or she does not have sufficient capacity to understand reasonably his or her condition, the nature and effect of proposed treatment, the risk of the treatment, and the consequences of no treatment. If a person has been declared legally incompetent by a previous court order, then that person is not capable of consenting to anything, including medical care. The designated guardian would be the appropriate decision maker. However, if the treatment is extraordinary or irreversible and would affect bodily integrity, then a court order must be sought for the procedure, rather than relying on the guardian's decision. If this means refusing or withdrawing life-sustaining treatment, state law generally will have specific provisions in its statutes and case law that must be followed.

Informed consent is a legal issue that often is taken for granted in the physician–patient relationship. It often is viewed as a form that must be signed before a procedure, when it really is about a discussion that must take place with the patient before delivering any care. However, as mentioned previously, it is the discussion that is fundamental to ensuring that the patient has sufficient information to make treatment choices that are right for him or her and to establishing a good relationship with the patient that will best protect a physician from claims of negligence.

MEDICAL RECORD PRACTICES

The HIPAA privacy regulations now govern the release of medical documentation, except that state law governs when it is stricter than the

HIPAA regulations. The health care provider is still the legal owner of patient medical records, but the information in the record is owned by the patient.

Documentation

The importance of accurate, objective, medical documentation cannot be overemphasized. As with patient communication, good documentation is central to providing quality medical care. It also is necessary for billing, proper insurance filing, and disability and workers' compensation claims and, of course, plays a major role in the event of litigation. The medical record has been characterized as a health professional's best friend or worst enemy, and has been described as the plaintiff attorney's "weapon of choice." During litigation or in working with dissatisfied patients prelitigation, good medical documentation will provide one of the most valuable assets to a defense against allegations of medical malpractice. A few guidelines for good documentation are as follows:

Maintain objectivity—keep the information as objective as possible, refrain from personal remarks about the patient, do not use the medical record to note disagreements with other medical professionals regarding patient care, avoid excessive adjectives and state the facts only.

Date, time, and sign notes—chronology often is important in investigating and assessing a case.

Write legibly.

Late notes should be identified as such; do not attempt to pass information added to the medical record as having been written at an earlier time.

Errors should be corrected by a single line drawn through the error; obliteration of errors is inadvisable when making corrections.

Show a thought process—the reasoning behind treatment or medication orders should be evidenced in the medical record. This is especially important when a treatment plan is altered from the original course of treatment.

Attribute quotes to the speaker so that such quotations are not reflected in the medical record as facts.

Document telephone calls—telephone contacts are the least likely to be documented in a medical record and yet may be crucial to constructing a chronology of patient care.

WHAT A PHYSICIAN SHOULD KNOW ABOUT MEDICAL MALPRACTICE INSURANCE

Obtaining adequate professional liability insurance is important to every physician and their group practice. There are two basic types of medical professional coverage. The traditional type, occurrence coverage, is very difficult to obtain in the marketplace today. Occurrence coverage provides funding for claims that arise out of a given policy year, regardless of the year that the claim actually is made. Thus, if you purchase occurrence coverage for each year that you are in practice, when you retire or change practice groups you will not have past claims that are uninsured (ie, no "tail" coverage is required). Unfortunately, insurers have found occurrence coverage difficult to price accurately, and thus are reticent to offer this type of coverage. Even when it is available, occurrence coverage generally is quite a bit more expensive than is the alternative, claims made coverage. However, because occurrence coverage leaves no tail to be funded later, if it is reasonably available, it is the preferred coverage to have.

The usual coverage available in the marketplace today is claims made coverage. This coverage provides funding for claims that are made during a given policy year, but that actually may have occurred in an earlier year. In other words, the insurer must cover you for when the claim actually is made. As a result, any time you change insurers, change employers, or retire, there are potential claims that already may have occurred but for which no claim has been made yet. As a result, any time you change insurers, change employers, or retire, you must purchase tail coverage from that insurer (or prior acts coverage from the new company who will cover you). Although claims made insurance is usually less expensive than is occurrence coverage on a year-to-year basis, it is necessary to purchase tail coverage as well. The cost of tail coverage varies from insurer to insurer and this formula also may change significantly from the time you first are insured by a company to the point at which you are retiring or otherwise making a change that requires the purchase of tail coverage. Tail coverage rarely is paid by your employer, but rather most often is the responsibility of the individual insured physician. It is very important that you plan for the cost of this coverage as you plan for retirement, change employers, or decide to switch insurance companies.

Also, when examining options for professional liability coverage, you also should pose the following questions and factor in the responses when choosing a company to provide this important coverage:

What is the financial stability of this medical malpractice insurer?

How long has the company been writing coverage in my state and can I expect them to continue to do so?

What are the limits of liability coverage being offered and what are the most appropriate limits for a family physician with my type of practice in my geographic practice area?

Who will pay the premium for the coverage—is it paid by me as the covered physician, or my employer?

Who will pay for any tail coverage and under what circumstances, if any? (On occasion, the employer will pay if they terminate your employment rather than vice versa or if you are retiring.)

Do I have a right to approve any settlement before it is agreed on?

Do I have a voice in selecting defense counsel? (Most often you will agree with the insurer because they have great interest in using good defense counsel, but you will want to know that you can request a change if the assigned counsel does not seem to be working out for one reason or another.)

Are punitive damages covered or excluded from coverage? (If excluded, you should have some idea as to how often they have been awarded in the area in which you are practicing.)

Are there other significant exclusions from coverage? (If so, you should have a good understanding of what those exclusions are and how common that type of exclusion is, as well as the risk of such a claim to you.)

Purchasing professional liability coverage is a significant expense of your practice of medicine. It also provides significant financial protection of your personal assets, so you should understand as much as possible about your coverage.

Key Points

- The focus on quality of care issues and patient safety will persist for the near future. Since the IOM published its first report, there have been numerous stories in the press and numerous publications that focus the public eye on medical errors and patient safety. These reports also have brought increased scrutiny of medical practices from state and federal government. Moreover, large employers who pay for the largest portion of health care in this country through employer-sponsored health insurance also have joined this quality initiative. The practice of medicine will feel the impact of this scrutiny through demands for the increased use of information technology, while also seeing increased regulations of medicine from government oversight bodies, and seeing payment for services increasingly tied in a variety of ways to patient outcomes.
- Patient confidentiality and privacy is a basic right that now is predicated on specific legal regulations under federal law. The federal government's privacy regulations are intended to create a minimum level of confidentiality for patient's health information across all states. Although the federal regulations do not create a private right for patient's to sue for breach of confidentiality, they may well establish the standard of care that courts may apply to future confidentiality claims. Understanding the patient's privacy rights and the physician's obligations under these regulations is imperative for the physician and for all those working in a physician's office.
- Establishing a patient relationship almost always is a choice of the physician, but once established, the relationship may not be terminated except within certain legal parameters. As a general rule, a physician does not have a duty to accept anyone as a patient. However, once a physician sees and examines a patient and agrees to treat him or her, the physician–patient relationship is established. There is then a duty to treat the patient until the condition that prompted the patient to see the physician is resolved

or until the relationship has been terminated appropriately within the constricts of the law. If the patient relationship is terminated inappropriately, the physician risks a claim of abandonment by the patient.
- Above all else, patients desire good communication with their physicians. Good rapport and communication with patients and their families is fundamental to good risk management in the practice of medicine. Patients who feel that they have not been listened to or feel that they did not understand what happened in their care are most likely to sue their physician. The informed consent process in a patient's care is a key opportunity to establish good communication. It is imperative that your practice establishes protocols for communicating important information about a patient's care to the patient and, when appropriate, to other involved health care providers.
- If you did not document it, outsides will often say it did not happen. The importance of accurate, objective, medical documentation cannot be overemphasized. As with patient communication, good documentation is central to providing quality medical care. In litigation, the medical record may become a physician's best friend or worst enemy, and has been described as a plaintiff attorney's "weapon of choice." It is essential that medical documentation be accurate, timely, and objective to be most credible.

References

[1] Black HC, editor. Black's law dictionary. 5th edition. St. Paul (MN): West Publishing Company; 1979.
[2] Novik R. Medical malpractice. February 19, 1995.
[3] Continuing medical malpractice insurance crisis. Hearing before the Subcommittee on Health of the Community of Labor and Public Welfare, 94th Congress, 1st Session, 154, 220.
[4] Kohn LT, Corrigan JM, Donaldson MS, editors. To err is human, building a safer health system. Washington, DC: National Academy Press; 2000.
[5] Hippocratic Oath. Webster's new universal unabridged dictionary, deluxe 2nd edition. Cleveland: Dorset & Baber; 1979.
[6] Bottrell MM, Alpert H, Fischbaum RL. Hospital informed consent for procedure forms: facilitating quality patient interaction. Arch Surg 2000;135:26–33.

Address reprint requests to

Rebecca W. West, MD
Piedmont Liability Trust
1020 Ednam Center, Suite 100
Charlottesville, VA 22903

e-mail: rww4q@virginia.edu

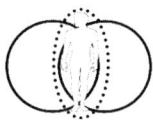

PROFESSIONAL AND PRACTICE MANAGEMENT SKILLS 1522–5720/03 $15.00 + .00

MEDICAL–LEGAL ISSUES: WHAT YOU SHOULD KNOW ABOUT THE LEGAL PROCESS

Rebecca W. West, JD

Most physicians want to avoid dealing with the litigation system, if possible. However, the likelihood of having to respond to the courts in some capacity periodically during your career is significant. If you are fortunate, you will never interface with the courts as a defendant. You are likely, however, to have to respond to subpoenas for records or your appearance at a deposition or trial, most often in the capacity of a treating physician of someone involved in the lawsuit. On occasion, you even may choose to act as an expert witness for your peers. It is important to understand the nature of the involved legal processes and how you might be expected to interface with the legal system.

THE LEGAL PROCESS

The Process for a Medical Malpractice Lawsuit

Service of Process

A Complaint or Motion for Judgment is filed in a state court, or a Complaint is filed in federal court. These suit papers then are served on the defendants, usually by a sheriff in the locale in which the defendant resides. You may be served anywhere—at home, at work, on a street corner—wherever the sheriff finds you. Service of process may be accepted by anyone else, at home or elsewhere, but that person will have

From the Piedmont Liability Trust, Charlottesville, Virginia; and the University of Virginia School of Medicine, Charlottesville, Virginia
Portions of this article are drawn from material previously produced by Ms. West for the Piedmont Liability Trust, Charlottesville, Virginia. The material is reprinted with permission of the Piedmont Liability Trust.

to sign as accepting the suit papers on your behalf. If someone else accepts service and signs for the lawsuit papers, it generally is seen the same as service of the papers on you personally. You should be certain that your office staff knows how legal papers served on you should be handled.

Court Pleadings

The heading of the lawsuit will tell you in which court the lawsuit is filed. It will then set forth the name of the plaintiff versus the name of the defendant. Once the lawsuit is filed in the court, it will be served on you, often by your local sheriff's office. In federal court, the lawsuit may be serviced by federal marshals or by federal process servers.

It is critical that you immediately are aware of any lawsuit, or other court order, served on you. Your response to a lawsuit must be filed with the court within the time frame set by your state law (most often within 21 days after you were served). If a response is not filed in this time frame, then a default judgment may be entered against you.

After the initial lawsuit is served on you, further pleadings and interaction between the plaintiffs and defendants must be through the attorneys. It is inappropriate for a defendant to call a plaintiff or vice versa.

Discovery

After suit has been filed and you have filed your initial response, discovery will ensue. The discovery process provides an opportunity to investigate the plaintiff's claim and the defendant's responses. The initial step in the discovery process is to file interrogatories, which are written questions answered under oath. Your attorney will send these interrogatories to you and give you a deadline for returning them. Your answers will be reviewed by your attorney, who may discuss them with you further, leading to revisions. The final answers must be by you and notarized. These answers may be amended later if need be; however, should you not amend them and your answers differ later in a deposition or at trial, these interrogatory responses may be used to attack your credibility. The interrogatory also will ask you to identify all witnesses for the defense, including experts and their expected opinions to be testified to at trial. The number and detail of questions will vary from case to case and from attorney to attorney. There may be questions that your attorney instructs you not to answer based on a legal objection. Your attorney also will pose interrogatories to the other side.

In addition to interrogatories, the plaintiff's attorneys may request you to produce documents. Your attorney may make legal objections to this request on your behalf.

Depositions are one of the most important tools of the discovery process. In addition to the parties to the lawsuit, all witnesses, expert or general, may be deposed. Generally, questions come only from the attorney on the opposing side. Your attorney will not want to reveal information or strategy for your defense so his or her questions will be reserved for trial. The deposition usually is relatively informal. Objections to questions are made but reserved for argument later if the matter goes to trial. On occasion, the issue is so important that the matter may be taken to the judge during or shortly after the deposition. However, in general, during a deposition, attorneys will make their objections and then instruct you to answer anyway. Again, the objections will be preserved on the record for later argument, if necessary. Although procedurally a deposition is informal, the importance of it cannot be underestimated because the answers given to questions at the deposition may be used to impeach a witness at trial if answers differ.

It may take a period of years to complete discovery. Once completed, a case may proceed to trial. Unlike old television stereotypes, the purpose of discovery is to reveal as much of the evidence as possible, and to avoid any surprises at trial. In many cases, the plaintiff will decide to withdraw the lawsuit, or the case will be settled before trial.

Trial

At trial, the plaintiff has the burden of proving his or her case by the greater weight (preponderance) of the evidence. The jury will decide if this burden is met, which means that they must find that it is greater than 50% likely that the negligence alleged actually occurred.

Before a trial begins, the selection of the jury, *voir dire*, occurs. In a civil case, there generally are seven jurors. The trial begins with the opening statement of the attorney for the plaintiff, followed by the opening statement of the defendant. The opening statements are not evidence, but rather are a preview of what the attorneys expect to present to the jury.

The plaintiff is first to put on his or her case. Witnesses called by the plaintiff are questioned first by plaintiff counsel. The plaintiff may not ask leading questions during this direct examination, such as "Isn't it true that...." On cross-examination by opposing counsel, leading questions may, however, be used. Giving short, concise answers that are responsive only to the question asked helps to avoid being boxed into an opinion or admission that you did not intend. Asking for questions to be clarified or repeated also is appropriate and helpful. You want to look at the attorney when he or she is asking a question, then turn and look at the jury when answering the question. At the completion of the plaintiff's evidence, the defendant may move the court to dismiss the plaintiff's case (a motion to strike by the defendant), if a *prima facie* case (the elements) has not been established.

It is rare for the defendant's motion to strike to be granted. Rather, the trial will move on to the defendant's evidence, which will seek to rebut the evidence introduced by the plaintiff. New evidence also may be introduced in an effort to provide an alternate theory of what occurred.

At the close of the defendant's evidence, the plaintiff has one last opportunity to put forth evidence that rebuts the defendant's case. Testimony by these rebuttal witnesses must be confined to contradicting evidence of the defendant.

Before deliberation by the jury begins, three more events will take place. First, the defendant again may move the court to have the case dismissed based on the plaintiff's failure to establish his or her case. Second, counsel will submit jury instructions to the judge who will select from those submitted as he or she deems appropriate. The instructions will be read to the jury by the judge before they enter their deliberations. The last information provided to the jury is the closing statements of counsel. Again, this is not evidence, but rather summations of the evidence presented in the light most favorable to the client. Plaintiff counsel's closing is first, and again the plaintiff gets a short period of time after the defense counsel's closing for rebuttal argument. This means that the last word to the jury will be from the plaintiff.

Jury deliberation may last a few minutes, a few hours, or even days. At this point there is nothing to do but wait.

Appeal

The plaintiff or defendant may appeal a case. Generally, there must be a legal basis for appeal rather than an appeal based on merits. It is possible, although very rare, that an appeal may be granted because there is a reasonable question that the jury's decision was not supported by the evidence. Because the courts give extreme deference to the jury, the likelihood of overturning the decision on this basis is slim. Most often, appeal is based on a mistake of law by the trial court judge. Should appeal be granted, a brief would be filed on the legal arguments, one from each side, with the plaintiff having the usual last retort. In addition, the appellate judges usually will hear oral arguments by the attorneys. No witnesses are introduced. The arguments are based on evidence and events in the trial court. The appellate court may decide that there is no basis for appeal, remand the case for retrial in the lower court with instructions on the applicable law, or dismiss the case altogether. How many levels of appeal there are depends on the particular state in which the case is being heard or whether it is in federal court.

The "Don'ts"

Don't Discuss the Case with Anyone Except Counsel

A lawsuit undoubtedly will evoke a variety of emotional responses and may tempt you to discuss your care with various people. Don't! In particular, do not contact the patient, the patient's family, or the patient's attorney. If treatment is continuing, avoid discussing any matters pertaining to the alleged malpractice and consult with your attorney regarding the advisability of transferring the patient's care to a colleague. Similarly, do not discuss the claim or the underlying facts with other health care providers, even if they also are named in the suit or provided care to the patient. Your attorney should be the person to contact all witnesses.

Don't Change the Records

Nothing can be more harmful to your case than for the plaintiff's attorney to find out that you have altered the records after receiving a lawsuit or a notice of a patient's intent to file a claim. Even a minor alteration (like correcting an obvious transcription error) will seriously hurt your credibility.

Don't Accept Calls From Other Attorneys

Once you are represented by counsel, the plaintiff's and codefendant's attorneys are prohibited from contacting you directly. All attempts by attorneys to contact you should be referred immediately to your attorney.

THE STANDARD OF CARE IN MEDICAL MALPRACTICE CASES

A claim of medical malpractice most commonly is based on the tort of negligence. To establish a doctor's negligence, the patient must prove four elements: (1) the doctor had a duty to the patient to conform to a specific standard of care, (2) the doctor breached that duty, (3) the doctor's breach was the actual and proximate cause of the patient's injury, and (4) the patient suffered damage from the breach.

The Standard of Care

The scope of the physician's duty to the patient is known as the "standard of care." The standard of care to which a physician generally is held is that degree of skill and diligence practiced by a reasonably prudent practitioner in the field of practice or specialty. As a general rule, a physician will be held to a statewide standard of care. That is, he or she will be expected to know and to provide the degree of care and skill possessed and exercised by doctors in the same field of practice or specialty throughout your state. Some states, however, apply a national standard of care. The standard of care is not intended to make the physician "an insurer of the success of his diagnosis and treatment" nor does it require the physician to provide "the highest degree of care known to his profession. The mere fact that he has failed to effect a cure or that his diagnosis and treatment have been detrimental to the patient's health does not raise a presumption of negligence" [1].

Establishing the Standard

Expert testimony ordinarily is necessary to establish the applicable standard of care. In most cases, the plaintiff is required to produce expert testimony that the defendant physician's conduct was not in accordance with customary practice. Failure to do so generally will result in dismissal of the lawsuit. The principal exceptions to this rule are sexual battery, lack of informed consent and foreign body cases in which malpractice is presumed and the burden shifts to the physician to prove that he or she did not act improperly.

A party cannot substitute medical books and treatises for the testimony of an expert witness. Such written evidence is hearsay and thus is inadmissible to prove the truth of the author's opinion. However, the expert can refer to and corroborate his or her testimony by such writings.

This same rule applies to the admission of medical equipment manuals and medical pamphlets, brochures, or instruction sheets published by drug manufacturers. Such writing generally is inadmissible to prove that the information contained in it is true, but it may be admissible to show simply that it existed and that the doctor should have known that it existed.

Similarly, practice parameters developed by national medical societies and other organizations generally are inadmissible to establish conclusively the standard of care. Such parameters, such as books and treatises, would be excluded as hearsay if offered as a truthful reflection of the standard of care. However, a medical expert can testify to and be cross-examined concerning a relevant parameter. The jury then can consider the guidelines in light of all the evidence, including the testimony of the expert witness. There appears to be an increase in the proffer of parameters by patients in the trials of medical malpractice actions.

Standards of care are not constant, but rather evolve and rise with the advent of new techniques, technologies, and medications. The physician is expected to stay current on these developments and to conform to generally accepted norms of medical practice.

SUBPOENAS

A witness also may be subpoenaed to appear at trial, when the trial is located in the same state as the witness. If the trial is outside of the state in which you, the witness, reside, you cannot be forced to appear at trial. Nonetheless, your deposition may be taken under subpoena earlier and then introduced at trial. Should you be subpoenaed to trial, you have a right to be paid a statutory witness fee and reasonable travel expenses, as set forth in your state's laws. You do not have a right to be paid any additional sums unless you become an expert for one of the parties to the case.

Once served with a subpoena for a deposition or for trial, you must appear at the date, time, and location shown on the court-ordered subpoenaed. If the date, time, or location is inconvenient, the only possibility for change is by agreement of the attorney who requested the subpoena. Normally, the schedule of a witness may be accommodated when planning a deposition. However, if deadline for discovery is approaching or trial is imminent, counsel may not be very accommodating toward you. Generally, counsel who need your testimony will try to make the process as convenient as possible to ensure that you are a cooperative witness. Nothing, however, requires counsel to change the subpoena date, time, or location. If you have been served with the subpoena and no changes have been agreed on by counsel, you must appear as required by law under the subpoena. Physicians have been sanctioned by courts for failing to respond to a subpoena.

It is worth noting that if you are subpoenaed for trial, the subpoena usually will give the first day of the trial. Many trials last for more than 1 day. You are under a continuing obligation to be present until you have been called to testify. However, most often the attorney subpoenaing you will tell you that you need not appear until a specific day and time when you are expected to be called to testify. If the attorney does not provide you with a specific day and time, you must appear on the day and at the time listed in the subpoena and remain throughout until you are dismissed by the court or the attorney who subpoenaed you.

If you have been served inappropriately with a subpoena (it is a case of mistaken identity or some privilege precludes your testimony), a motion to quash the subpoena must be filed in advance of the time you are commanded to appear. The motion must be filed in the court in which the lawsuit is being heard. The court most likely will set a hearing on the motion to quash the subpoena. As the subpoenaed witness, you may be required to present evidence to the court, or the court may choose to rely on information presented by counsel. If the court overrules the motion to quash, then you must appear as required by the subpoena.

When subpoenaed as a witness, as opposed to an expert witness, you are required to give testimony only about information directly related to your involvement in the matter that is the subject of the lawsuit. For example, in the instance in which there is a personal injury lawsuit arising out of an automobile accident, if you are called as a treating physician, you need only testify as to the actual treatment you rendered or the medical opinion you reached at the time of treatment. You should not render an opinion about the long-term effects of the person's injuries unless you reached those conclusions at the time of treatment, nor should you give an opinion on the cause of the injuries unless you reached that opinion at the time of treatment, based on sufficient information to allow you to reach that conclusion. These types of questions call for expert testimony, which you have not been paid to give and you cannot, under the usual circumstances, be required to give.

If an attorney in a case wishes for you to testify as an expert witness when you were a treating physician, generally the court will allow this. There have been instances in which courts have found it inappropriate for a treating physician to testify as an expert. Assuming that the court will allow it, it is worth considering whether you wish to accept the role as an expert witness. It is purely voluntary whether you accept this role. However, if you are a treating physician who is required to testify, you may wish to consider being designated as an expert witness, assuming there are no conflicts that would preclude this. By choosing to act as an expert, you ensure some compensation for the time and inconvenience of your involvement in the lawsuit. Once you agree to act as an expert, counsel who retained you reasonably may expect you to do additional preparation so that opinion questions can be answered with credibility. However, if called as a general witness, there is no requirement that you do anything to prepare for your deposition or for the trial. You are not required to have reviewed the medical records and should not do medical research on issues regarding the patient. (As a general witness, you are not being paid to do this work, nor are you being qualified by the court as an expert to give opinions.) Reviewing the patient's medical records and being generally familiar with the patient's care, however, usually will make your testimony go more quickly.

Let's look at several instances in which you may receive a subpoena and your obligations in those circumstances. If you receive a *subpoena duces tecum* (a subpoena for records), you are being required to produce only records. Under this subpoena, you need appear only if you do not produce the demanded records on or before the date stated in the subpoena. If you believe that there is some reason not to disclose the records, you may choose to contact the patient to ensure that he or she is aware of the subpoena for his or her records. It is then incumbent upon the patient to have their attorney file a motion with the court to quash the subpoena. The Health Insurance Portability and Accountability Act (HIPAA) also has created a new duty, which requires that the attorney serving the subpoena notify any patient whose records have been subpoenaed and give the patient an opportunity to file a motion to quash. Your state's laws may dictate exactly how this process works; however, you may not release records, even under subpoena, until the HIPAA and your state law requirements have been satisfied.

If you receive a subpoena in a child abuse case in which you were a treating physician, most likely you will be called by the state's attorney. You are not being called as an expert witness, but rather as a general witness and have a right only to receive the witness fee and expenses. The subpoena generally will be to appear in a court that is assigned to deal with juvenile or domestic relations matters. Usually, you will not have an option to change the date or time you have been subpoenaed to appear. When several treating clinicians have been subpoenaed, the attorney may agree to simply call one or two of those involved to testify. On rare occasions, an agreement may be reached to conduct your testimony in the hearing by telephone. Any such accommodations are purely discretionary with the attorney and cannot be imposed no matter how inconvenient it is to appear in court.

It also has become more common for treating physicians to be subpoenaed as witnesses to testify in child custody or domestic dispute cases. In most instances, the attorney will contact you ahead of time to ask that you act as an expert. If, however, you receive a subpoena to appear, it may well be to testify as a treating physician and general witness for which you will not be paid.

It is never appropriate to talk to an attorney by phone or in person or even to release patient records to the attorney unless you have the patient's HIPAA compliant authorization to do so or unless there is a court order for you to do so.

THE STRESS OF LITIGATION

A phenomenon known as Litigation Stress Syndrome is encroaching on the lives of physicians and other health care professionals. Dr. Sara Charles and Dr. Edward Reading were the first to recognize the syndrome in which individuals named in a malpractice claim experience stress-related reactions. The onset may be immediate, with the individual experiencing feelings of isolation and anger and a questioning of his or her ability and self-worth. In most individuals, however, the process is gradual, reflected in a depressed mood, insomnia, frustration, and the emergence of physical symptoms [2].

In her pioneer studies, Dr. Charles found that 39.1% of Cook County Illinois physicians who were sued reported experiencing "major depressive disorder" [2]. Twenty-six percent of those physicians had symptoms for more than 2 weeks. More than 20% of the physicians felt pervasive anger with a multitude of other problems such as inner tension, irritability, insomnia, fatigue, headache, and gastrointestinal symptoms. An exacerbation of a preexisting health disorder was another likely response to the physician being named in a claim [2].

Additional symptoms that may emerge include those that are personal in nature: alcohol and drug abuse, emotional volatility, fatigue, family and marital problems, depression, insecurity, frustration, and anxiety. Psychosomatic disorders, eating disorders, suicide ideation, and acts of violence also may arise. The organizational symptoms that have been identified include reduced productivity, increased errors, absenteeism, premature retirement, and impaired decision making.

The filing of a medical malpractice claim usually triggers Litigation Stress Syndrome, with stress escalating as the claim progresses. The "peaks and valleys" of the medical malpractice process tend to add to the stress. There are peak periods of claims activity that make it necessary for the practitioner to increase the time spent with his or her lawyer, whether to answer interrogatories or prepare for a deposition. Perhaps more difficult is the adjustment to the "valleys"—the periods during which no activity occurs, and the practitioner cannot force the issues and bring closure.

G. B. Patrick [3] has described five phases of Litigation Stress Syndrome that are not unlike the stages of grief. These phases are

1. Denial ("I did my best for my patient and why me"?)
2. Anger ("How dare I be accused of malpractice.")

3. Bargaining ("If I get through this I promise to be an even better health care practitioner.")
4. Depression ("This is only going to get worse.")
5. Acceptance ("I will get through this.")

Risk managers are developing strategies to assist health care professionals in dealing with litigation stress. Stress management programs have been created to provide education and support to physicians, nurses, and other health care practitioners who are named in malpractice claims [3].

Litigation stress support groups and other self-help groups may come together to educate practitioners about the litigation process and to assist them in developing coping skills. J. Pfifferling has suggested ground rules for the establishment of litigation stress management support groups [4]:

Confidentiality
Participants refrain from advice giving
Discussion is oriented around professional problems that affect the individual personally or socially
Only subjects that are agreeable to individual members are pursued
Meeting termination times are established and followed
No psychologic labeling is used
No visitors are allowed unless the group members unanimously agree

To protect these group discussions from plaintiff discovery attempts, neither your specific case, nor the cases of others cases, should be discussed.

CHOOSING AN ATTORNEY

As discussed above, if you are sued for medical malpractice, your insurer generally will assign and pay for your attorney. Because insurers regularly engage attorneys to defend claims, you should consider the insurer to have the best interest of the case in mind when selecting an attorney to represent you. Recognize that medical malpractice cases, on average, take 5 years to be resolved. Thus, you will be dealing with the case and the attorney over years. As a result, you want to be sure that you are comfortable with the attorney. You also want to be sure that you do not have unrealistic expectations of your attorney. There will be periods of time when you may hear from your attorney often, such as when you are preparing for your deposition or the depositions of other key witnesses or when your are preparing for trial. There will be other long periods during which you may hear nothing from your attorney because no significant activities are taking place. However, you should be comfortable requesting a status report from your attorney at any time. Most often the attorney will not contact you when he or she has nothing new to report.

Never hesitate to question your attorney with regard to the handling of your case if you have concerns. Although the attorney is paid by the insurance company, his or her ethical duty is first and foremost to your defense. The attorney has an ethical duty to apprise you of any probable conflicts of interest between you and the insurance company. For instance, if there is a reasonable chance that a verdict could be rendered that exceeds the amount of your insurance coverage, you may have personal exposure that suggests you consider hiring a personal attorney (paid for by you) to advise you on the risk over and above your insurance coverage. Ultimately, if you believe that your attorney is handling your case in a manner deemed inappropriate, you should contact your insurance company and discuss your concerns and question whether a different attorney should be assigned.

There basically are four other areas of law in which you might anticipate engaging an attorney. Each area of practice is different, most often necessitating that different attorneys be retained to handle each area. Generally, you will want to hire an attorney who concentrates his or her practice in the needed area. If you are setting up your medical practice; negotiating your employment contract with a practice, hospital, or other health care company; or buying, reorganizing, or selling a practice you will want to retain atransactional health care lawyer whose practice regularly includes these types of issues. If you have financial questions that bear on either personal or business tax matters, you most likely will want to contact your accountant first. If there are concerns or unanswered questions, then turn to a tax attorney. If a third party is challenging you on tax issues on other personal or business finance issues, then you should engage an attorney to assist you specifically with regard to those matters being challenged. For personal financial planning, most physicians will want to consult an estate planning attorney as their career matures or they prosper.

Each of the noted areas of law generally requires an attorney with experience and special knowledge in the matters at hand. However, when doing personal real estate transactions or small claims collection, an attorney in the general practice of law often is adequate. A general practice attorney also may be able to assist with simple criminal issues such as traffic violations or simple divorce proceedings. Regardless of the issues, you should feel comfortable asking the attorney up front what his or her relevant experience is, and have a clear understanding at the outset of what the attorney's fees will be, and how and when you will be billed for services. When hiring an attorney, it is reasonable to rely on the recommendations of peers, friends, or family members; but you also should do your own due diligence with regard to the attorney's background and suitability for your particular legal needs.

SUMMARY

The manner in which physicians interface with the law in their daily practice of medicine varies greatly. The need to be informed of legal issues arising in one's practice has become essential. It also has meant that the

---

Key Points

- In providing care to patients, from a legal standpoint, physicians will be held to the standard of care of what a reasonably prudent physician in the same or similar field or specialty would have done under the same or similar circumstances. Negligence is the most common basis for a medical malpractice lawsuit. To establish negligence in most malpractice cases, a claimant must establish that the defendant physician breached the standard of care. The standard of care is established by testimony of an expert witness from the same or similar field or specialty who testifies to a reasonable degree of medical certainty what should have been done under the same or similar circumstances. A jury then will decide what experts they find to be most credible in making a finding with regard to a defendant physician's liability. Without the testimony of a peer stating that you breached the standard of care, it is rare that for a plaintiff to prevail on a claim of medical malpractice.
- A subpoena is a court order with which a physician must comply once the subpoena has been served. Should you be subpoenaed to trial or a deposition, you have a right to be paid a statutory witness fee and reasonable travel expenses as set forth by applicable state laws. You do not have a right to be paid any additional sums unless you become an expert for one of the parties in a case. Once served with a subpoena for a deposition or trial, you must appear at the date, time, and location shown on the court-ordered subpoena. When responding to a subpoena to produce a patient medical record or to be present at a deposition to respond to questions with regard to your care of a patient, federal privacy regulations stipulate a process that must be followed before releasing any information to a patient as mandated under the subpoena. Medical records should not be released until you or your staff has verified that the subpoena for records has met HIPAA privacy requirements.
- Being a defendant in a medical malpractice claim is stressful to involved physicians and their families. There is a recognized phenomenon known as Litigation Stress Syndrome. If you are involved in medical malpractice litigation, the stress of this lawsuit likely will affect you personally, as well as your family and your medical practice. Understanding the potential stress and working to manage its impact on you and those around you is essential.

---

breadth of knowledge your business managers for the practice must acquire has increased significantly. This means that educational materials to keep you up to date with legal issues are a necessary part of your practice. In addition, you will need to have a health care lawyer who is familiar with current medical–legal issues to whom you can turn when needed. This article has sought to provide a framework for some of the most common issues you may encounter in your daily practice.

References

[1] *Brown v Kaulizakis*, 229 Va. 524, 331 S.E.2d 440 (1985).

[2] Charles SC. Malpractice suits: their effects on doctors, patients and families. Journal of the Medical Association of Georgia 1987;76.
[3] Patrick GB. Small deaths: an editorial. ACMS Bulletin 1988:2.
[4] Wilbert JR, Charles SC, Reading E. Coping with the stress of malpractice litigation. Illinois Medical Journal 1987.

Address reprint requests to

Rebecca W. West, MD
Piedmont Liability Trust
1020 Ednam Center
Suite 100
Charlottesville, VA 22903

e-mail: rww4q@virginia.edu

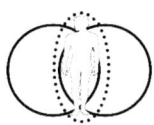
PROFESSIONAL AND PRACTICE MANAGEMENT SKILLS 1522–5720/03 $15.00 + .00

HEALTH INSURANCE SYSTEMS FOR FAMILY PHYSICIANS

Kyle L. Grazier

Insurance is a mechanism to protect individuals or groups against loss. Insurance has a long and storied history over centuries. Some accounts have dated the original practice of insurance to the Babylonian era, when traders were paid contingent on the safe delivery of goods, and the first insurance contract the shipping industry of fourteenth-century Europe. As part of British marine practices in the eighteenth century, individuals would sign their names and the level of risk they were willing to assume at the bottom of the risk contract—thus, introducing the term "underwriting," which still is used today to describe the acceptance or rejection of risk by an insurer. In the nineteenth century, US federal and state governments—seeing the catastrophic losses resulting from floods, droughts, and fires—began offering property and casualty, crop, life, and eventually disability and sickness insurance to communities. In addition, governments began to mandate the maintenance of financial reserves by employers or contractors to help absorb the losses incurred by citizens.

In the late 1800s, friendly and benevolent societies offered sickness and disability insurance, some of the first-recorded contracts dealing specifically with health services coverage polices similar to those of today. In the mid-1900s, unions and employers began to offer health insurance benefits to workers; benefits often were used to attract labor when wages were frozen or labor was scarce [1].

Relative to the practice of medicine, health insurance is a young field. Even more recent is the impact of health care coverage and its administration on the daily practice of medicine, both clinically and operationally.

THE ROLE OF HEALTH INSURANCE

In the United States, the vast majority of individuals with health insurance are covered by private rather than public plans. Although

From the Department of Health Management and Policy, School of Public Health, University of Michigan, Ann Arbor, Michigan national health insurance has been discussed since the 1930s, as yet, no comprehensive publicly financed and delivered program exists that meets the needs now addressed by private insurers. The extent to which insurance is used as a means to redistribute resources among the sick and healthy and those who can and cannot pay is based on tenets of "distributive justice."

Stone [2] contends that actuarial fairness dictates medical underwriting, or segmenting of risks based on health status. They argue that underwriting, used by many traditional insurers, fragments communities into smaller and smaller groups; the cost of services used is borne by those in the group. Before long, the price of insurance for that small group of high users exceeds what they can afford, and the group becomes unable to pay for insurance or care.

Alternatively, under a social insurance model, the amount paid for coverage is not tied to individual medical need or ability to pay. In reviewing the insurance contracts discussed in this article, it behooves the physician or analyst to examine how closely allied the particular insurance processes and products are with these philosophies and the outcome of those assumptions.

Medicine recognizes the variation in health status within populations and the fact that demand for care correlates, although not perfectly, with medical need. Andersen's model of health use [3,4] is one of the best known in health services research and provides some potential reasons for the variation in cases seen in the medical office. Briefly, in the Andersen model, health care use is a function of three independent characteristics of the individual: predisposing characteristics, such as gender and age; enabling characteristics, such as insurance coverage and income; and need characteristics, such as symptom patterns, severity of illness, and perceived health. Each dimension is hypothesized to exert an independent influence on services use, measured in a number of ways: number of visits, any use, number of hospitalizations, and other indicators of use. Health insurance recognizes this variation and capitalizes on it to charge a price, or premium, based on the expected use by the entire population. "Expected use" ties together the medical need for care, care-seeking behavior, and the expected costs of that care; in this way, insurance spreads the risk of medical need and economic loss across those who do and do not seek services and those who can and cannot pay.

If large numbers of individuals avert risk, there is potential for this behavior to result in a reduction in the supply of care or high prices. If a provider cannot get paid for the resources consumed in delivering care, then financial viability is threatened. Eventually providers limit care to those who have the means to pay, leaving those who are poor and sick without care. The high chance of there being great economic loss from such a business discourages that business and, in the longer run, the medical care system collapses or is reconfigured in a less-optimal manner.

Because of the potential social and economic harm related to medical care risk, insurance is a heavily regulated business. The extent and type of regulation differ across forms of insurance; and, even for the same type of insurance, regulations differ across states. This lack of uniformity in state codes of insurance makes it more complex for companies to operate across states.

States regulate insurers who wish to offer or "write" insurance business within the state. Because predictors of future claims may not always be precise, states require insurers to maintain a fund, called a reserve, to ensure that the company can cover its promises to cover all losses that arise in the course of doing business in the state. Some states also regulate the administrative fees that can be imposed on customers. Because most insurers are for-profit firms and, in many cases, are traded publicly on a stock exchange, distribution of profits also is subject to regulation. Two forms of insurers exist in the United States—stock companies and mutual companies. These differ by who "owns" the company: those who buy shares of stock in the company ("stock" companies) and company policyholders who, by virtue of being covered by the company, also "own" the company (a "mutual" company). Profits are distributed accordingly.

MODELS OF HEALTH INSURANCE

Because health insurance in the United States is tied primarily to employment and health plans compete in the market for employers, details of the basic health insurance products differ significantly [5]. Models of coverage based on a charge set by a physician for a service and paid by the patient have been rare for some time. Pure health-maintenance organization (HMO)-based care, in which salaried doctors in HMO-owned facilities provide all the care at one site, is equally uncommon. Health care coverage arrangements that have some similarities to each of these models dominate the large group market. This heterogeneity imparts complexity and unintended incentives on health care delivery systems.

Two models—indemnity-type coverage and managed care networks—have emerged to encompass most of what physicians see among their patients with private health insurance. To "indemnify" is to compensate for a loss. Under an indemnity-type policy, the physician charges a fee for the service delivered and the patient pays the charge and then turns to the insurance plan for reimbursement. A schedule of benefits dictates the types of medical services for which payment can be expected—either in part or in full, directly or indirectly from the patient and insurer. The patient is charged a fee and the forms required to collect payment are submitted by the physician's office or by the patient for payment. The amount paid is based on the "usual and customary" payment amount, based on the rate for that procedure in the community in which the physician practices and the level negotiated with similar physicians who provide those services.

The managed care model is as broad in its actual practice as is the indemnity model of insurance. Managed care organizations and arrangements have been in existence for decades. Early in the nineteenth century, railroad, lumber, and some mining industries arranged for capitation arrangements with local physicians to provide services to their workers. Benevolent societies also provided prepaid health services as part of their membership benefits. In the twentieth century, prepaid group practices—or medical services plans, as they also were known—developed and proliferated to care for select groups of employees; later, they opened enrollment to other sectors of the public. Some prepaid group practices that are still in existence include Kaiser Permanente Health Plan, Group Health Cooperative of Puget Sound, and Health Insurance Plan of Greater New York, although they now have different corporate structures.

These and future managed care models sought to improve enrollees' access to services by dedicating providers and facilities to their care. From the provider viewpoint, patients seen in the office could be offered all and any care necessary to treat them, as long as care was furnished through the managed care organization. Although this model still exists in some markets, it has been modified along several dimensions.

Network model managed care arrangements have grown substantially in number of plans and in enrollment market share. In these arrangements, independent physicians contract with the managed care plan and negotiate arrangements to be paid either a monthly or annual fee per plan enrollee that is independent of use, or a discounted fee for services rendered. Enrollees in the managed care plans are restricted to plan-contracted providers for care, or receive services from the network providers at a lower cost than the care received from nonnetwork providers. Because of the potential incentives for physicians to undertreat those for whom a standard fee is received regardless of services sought, and for enrollees to overuse services that are at a lower cost to them, several utilization management processes are imposed on both the enrollees and the physicians. These management processes include controls over specialist use through mandatory referral processes and advanced review and approvals of high-cost services, new technology, and emergency room and hospital care. Managed care plans also have implemented disease-management programs to ensure that those who have chronic or severe illnesses receive the appropriate type and amount of care over the required time period.

PAYING FOR CARE

Historically, the provider's price for services was based on the costs of the care delivered. The physician priced standard services similarly and the patient was charged accordingly. However, individual patients and providers cannot singularly bear limitless medical and economic risk. Within the physicians' pool of patients there may be severely or chronically ill individuals and families. The physician practice may be located in an economically vulnerable area; with an economic downturn, patients may find themselves unable to pay for necessary care.

The purpose of insurance is to transfer or reduce risk. By spreading individual risks over large numbers of individuals, the probability of events that seem random can be estimated. Forecasting collective losses replaces forecasting the loss for any one individual. The responsibility for estimating these probabilities falls with the actuary. Using broad mathematic models, the actuary estimates the expected use of services and their costs, based on past use by the same groups of people or use by similar groups, for services sought under particular benefit coverage [6]. The actuary takes into account group attributes such as the age, gender, type of employment, and family size of the potential enrollees, as well as potential environmental determinants of use and cost, such as new medical technology, the economy, and potential disease exposures. It is the job of the underwriter to determine whether and how to apply the estimates produced by the actuary to a potential insurance customer. The underwriter determines how much weight to place on past use, demographic factors, or the stability of the workforce. By examining, accepting, or rejecting the potential risks of a client, the underwriter determines the profits the insurer will realize after paying claims and expenses.

There is some evidence that underwriting is subject to an "underwriting cycle," or a periodic and regular change in the competitiveness of the insurance product [7]. In the process of examining the loss ratios, or the ratio of premiums collected to losses incurred, underwriters may see years in which losses exceeded collections. As part of the cycle, underwriters then may tighten underwriting standards and charge higher premiums, bringing more profits to the industry; this, in turn, attracts more insurers and more capital. More insurers with higher profits increases competition for business, which, in turn, results in relaxed underwriting standards and lower premiums to gain business, eventually resulting in more losses than premiums. Such market activity forces some insurers out of the business, at which point underwriting standards again begin to tighten, continuing the cycle. Employers and others who offer health benefits may see the cycle reflected in the prices they are charged for insurance or in the competitiveness of the bids. This may explain, in part, why physicians will see variations over time in the stringency or generosity of the benefits available to their patients.

Because insurers rely, to a varying extent, on the enrollee characteristics and the past use by those enrollees, if enrollees know more about their needs and intentions to use services than the underwriting models would predict, insurers may be faced with unexpected losses. When information about the expected use of services differs between the insurer and the insured, two common problems associated with this information asymmetry arise: biased selection and moral hazard [8]. Biased selection can take the form of favorable or adverse selection; in either case, the insured intends to join one plan or another based on information that only the insured knows. In the case of adverse selection, the insured knows in advance of selecting a plan that there will be a higher than average use of services and selects the plan that will pay the most for those services [9]. Moral hazard exists in a simple form when the insurer does not know in advance the average cost of the risk. Once enrolled in the plan, a member may use excess services, over and above the level expected when the premium was set. These events result in skewed use of services by particular individuals and skewed costs to the plan or to the physician group.

From the physician's perspective, the distinctions between indemnity and managed care models and adverse selection and moral hazard impact the manner in which he or she is paid. If a physician participates in the managed care plan's network of approved providers, the amount, timing, and basis of payment depends on a negotiated arrangement between plan and physician. The parties negotiate a certain payment level per service or a lump sum payment per enrollee in the plan, regardless of the amount of service delivered to the patient. Patients with known needs for services who select into an indemnity-type plan may require services of a more intense nature and frequency; the administration of the indemnity policies with variable coverage often demand considerable administrative resources to assist patients in paying for and collecting reimbursement from the policies.

THE BUSINESS OF INSURANCE

The basic unit of insurance is the contract. Because this is a legally binding contract between insurer and insured, certain conditions of any legal contract are required. For instance, the contract is not valid unless there is consideration—which, in the case of an insurance contract, is not necessarily the up-front payment of premiums or services, but rather the promise to pay. The insurer gives consideration in the form of the promise to pay when the agreed-upon events occur. The insured gives consideration in the promise to pay premiums.

Insurance is considered an aleatory contract; both parties understand that the amount exchanged may not be equal. The insured may pay more in premiums than the insurer pays in losses. Commutative contracts presume that both parties contribute equally valued amounts to the contract. Because of the feature of chance, the insurance contract is considered aleatory. Insurance contracts also exceed the standards of usual contracts in their "utmost good faith" or *uberrimae fidi* basis, rather than the bona fide basis of most contracts. This higher standard translates to agreements by the insured, if asked, to share information on expected use—for example, information about a health condition—before enrolling in a plan. In this way, the insured does not have information that the insurer lacks to price the product fairly. The insurer also is held to a higher standard of good faith, in agreeing to reimburse or provide services promised under the contract. One of the purposes of state regulation of insurance is to ensure that this utmost good faith has sufficient financing behind it.

Property, liability, and most health insurance contracts are contracts of indemnity, which means that they compensate the insured only for those losses incurred. Under the principle of indemnity, there are three important doctrines [10]. The first principle is based on the notion that the insured must have an insurable interest in whatever is under contract. This means that for health insurance, the insured must be the subject, owner, and beneficiary of the insurance.

The second doctrine of indemnity is that there must be limitations in the contract that define the actual maximum amount of the liability or what the insurer will pay. For health insurance, this includes explicit information on coinsurance, copayments, and deductibles. Often some of the principles of indemnity are violated; in this circumstance, the underwriter has determined that a particular clause does not create a moral hazard.

Indemnity also gives the insurer the right of subrogation, the third doctrine that derives from indemnity. Under subrogation, the insurer has the right to collect payment for a loss incurred by the insured from a third party if the third party is responsible for the loss. For instance, if a health plan member incurs costs for medical care received due to a car accident, the health plan would cover that care, but then seek reimbursement from the driver who caused the accident. Subrogation is applied only against third parties.

Insurance contracts also are very specific about what is included in the standard coverage and what must be purchased separately under a "rider" to the policy. Riders are separate "mini-contracts" that can, for a fee, be added to the benefits provided under the primary contract. Riders are underwritten and priced separately from the standard coverage and often offer benefits that a particular employer may feel are particularly attractive to the employees or to the employer, but are nonstandard in contracts. Standard contract language addresses which losses are covered, such as medical expenses for inpatient care or outpatient surgery; which hazards are excluded, such as acts of war or accidents suffered in the military; whether deductibles apply to individuals and/or families; whether deductibles apply to particular medical conditions, and if so, which conditions; any maximums or limits on coverage and for what time period they are in force; and the level of "participation" or the proportion of the costs exceeding the deductible for which the insured must pay [10].

One critical distinction between the indemnity model and the HMO model is the manner in which the premium charged for the coverage is calculated. The extent to which each type of plan relies on the past experience of the covered members differs. For indemnity-type plans, premiums are set based on the actual claims experience of the population being insured, adjusted for expected cost increases, administrative costs, the amount of money required as a reserve fund for the insurer, and a factor for the credibility of the data and the forecasts [11,12]. For most managed care plans, "rating" of the coverage, or pricing it, depends on a community rate; this estimate of future costs is based on the entire population covered by the plan, adjusted for age and gender of the particular group of contract holders.

For those risks that exceed the levels deemed acceptable by the insurer, reinsurance companies offer contracts that insure the insurer. Reinsurers sell layers, or "trenches," of risk protection to the purchaser.

The primary insurer "cedes" the risk to the reinsurer in a process known as "cession." There are two basic types of reinsurance: treaty and facultative reinsurance. These distinctions are based on the contract drawn between the insurer and the reinsurer. Treaty contracts require far less negotiation at the time of loss, whereas a facultative contract offers options to both parties in the event of loss; these options include whether and at what level to give or accept coverage for the loss. Reinsurance can be purchased to cover aggregate or individual risks. For instance, an insurer or health plan might decide to reinsure for individual cases that exceed a certain claim cost level; alternatively it may choose to reinsure for claims costs that in total for the year exceed a certain level. Reinsurance plays a role in several aspects of the health insurance markets. Traditional indemnity insurers, HMOs, and employers who are self-funded and therefore bear the risk themselves may purchase reinsurance [13]. One common arrangement is to purchase reinsurance to cover 90% of the claims costs that exceeded 120% of the company's expected total claims costs for the year.

MEDICARE AND MEDICAID

Amendments in 1965 to the Social Security Act created Medicaid and Medicare. The intent was to provide mechanisms for providing physical and financial access to some medical services for some special populations. The political, social, and administrative histories of the programs have been written from many perspectives. Although at the time of their passage many dubbed the programs "national health insurance," Medicare is restricted to most Americans over 65, and, as of 1972, those disabled persons receiving cash benefits for 24 months under the Social Security program and those with end-stage renal disease. Medicaid is a federal–state program and as such varies significantly by state, beyond the basic restrictions imposed by the federal portion. Administratively, both programs currently are managed by the Centers for Medicare and Medicaid Services (CMS), formerly known as the Health Care Financing Administration. CMS is part of the Department of Health and Human Services, which also is responsible for other agencies and programs such as the National Institutes of Health and the Centers for Disease Control and Prevention.

Medicare is the largest health insurer in the United States. By covering many medical services for the majority of the aged, the government participates in a relatively high-risk, high-cost market. However, Medicare does not cover all costs of care. Private insurance is used to supplement the coverage and the payment provided by Medicare. Medicare supplemental policies, known as MediGap policies, are designed to cover payment for services such as the deductibles and copayments that are not covered under Medicare. If a Medicare beneficiary also is covered under an employer group health plan, services are paid first by that plan (the primary payer, or "primary to Medicare"), and, if those services are not paid for in full, the claim is sent to Medicare for payment of the remaining covered charges. These protocols for assigning responsibility for first and second payment generally are known as coordination of benefits (COB). COB attempts to ensure that the payment for services for which the patient has coverage are assigned to the proper payer; however, at no time is the payment to exceed the total charge incurred.

Because of the market power of Medicare, its policies touch almost every aspect of care delivery and payment. Other programs and insurers often replicate the methods designed by CMS to measure, reflect, and pay for resources. Payment models of physician, hospital, nursing home, home care, and outpatient care fees usually are pilot tested through government-sponsored demonstrations before widespread implementation, which normally is phased into use over a number of years.

One of the most significant models imposed by Medicare was its hospital payment system, passed into law in 1983. Use of diagnostic categories known as Diagnosis Related Groups (DRGs) replaced a cost-based system—albeit with controls on rates of increase and allowable costs—in existence in various forms for almost 2 decades. This prospective, case-based system theoretically recognized all of the resources attributed to the care of a Medicare patient in the hospital by assigning the proper DRG to the case. Payment was based on the DRG for the patient, representing the diagnosis that caused the admission, and limited to this amount. To avoid incentives to admit more patients (because payment was on a per-admission basis), Medicare also implemented more stringent protocols for monitoring activities, to help ensure that patients were not discharged too quickly under the plans. This prospective payment system had a mechanism for recognizing those cases that exceeded certain levels of cost that far exceeded the DRG payment built into it. This outlier policy was intended to reduce the tendency of hospitals to discharge too quickly, particularly those cases for which the DRG payment was deemed inadequate by the hospital. The outlier policies used by Medicare illustrate one method to reduce the risk to a hospital of an adverse and excessive loss [14]. By paying extra for those cases that are outliers, Medicare is, in principle and in practice, reinsuring the hospital for excessive loss [15].

Medicare also has played a significant role in the development of physician payment systems [16]. In an effort to measure and eventually pay for the resources used in delivering physician care, studies funded by the government measured the resources used in managing a clinical office, the time spent with the patient, and the time and resources required in the training and education of the physician [17]. These factors were analyzed and resulted in a relative resource-based scale of values assigned to procedures performed by the physician. A cost factor is determined annually by Medicare and assigned to the relative values for procedures, resulting in the payment amount received by the physician for the care.

Many physician practices use this same relative value scale structure as the basis for their primary billing practices. The relative weights assigned to the procedure codes can be accumulated for an individual physician or group of physicians and a constant or variable cost factor is applied to determine the charge for that service. The procedure codes can be weighted further for different diagnostic categories.

THE PROCESS OF INSURANCE

Understanding the administrative systems involved in handling insurance payments is important to a financially viable clinical office and to keeping patients satisfied. It also helps in understanding some of the pitfalls in pricing insurance.

Traditional indemnity and indemnity-like insurers use standardized electronic and paper forms to collect and process data for payment and record keeping. The data required for payment by government programs and private insurers constitute a "claim" and consist of patient and member identifiers such as name, Social Security number or unique member identifier, date of birth, address, and telephone number. Clinical data consists of dates of service, site of service, type of provider or provider identifier, procedures and diagnosis codes, and charge. The codes for procedures follow the Health Care Common Procedure Coding System, an alphanumeric coding system that includes the Current Procedural Terminology procedure codes used to describe a service. Diagnosis is recorded using the most recent International Classification of Diseases coding system. The diagnosis codes are organized by body system; the codes are three-numeric digits followed by a decimal point and one or more numeric "modifiers" for additional details about the disorder. For inpatient service records, the DRG code also is recorded. These claims data form the basis for individual payment, but also are used by insurers and data companies to estimate use and cost experience for groups.

Claims are considered "incurred" upon delivery of the service. When the claim is submitted to the insurer and recorded in their system, it is considered "reported." Claims that are incurred but not yet reported (IBNR) to the insurer or health plan can make it difficult to track accurately the liabilities of the insurer at any particular time. Estimates of the extent of the IBNR claims are incorporated into most prospective premium calculations.

The Actuarial Standards Board recommends certain practices when using claims data [18]. They recognize that for health actuaries to estimate incurred health claims, develop rates, and analyze and project trends, claims data may be the best and most reliable source. However, failure to recognize how certain business practices and benefit plan provisions affect the frequency, severity, and cost of claims can lead to estimates that may not reflect actual use under a different set of benefit designs and premium levels. The type and level of benefit, including restrictions and copayments, influence how services are used. Benefits, economic circumstances, provider fee changes, and catastrophic events affect the types and timing of claims incurred.

SUMMARY

In the United States, the practice of medicine is linked to the practice of insurance. The language and processes of paying for care permeate the delivery of services. The connection between needing health care and having it available is mediated by a complex system of risk assessment, estimation, and pricing. For family physicians to deliver their services, a basic understanding of who pays and how they pay is essential [19]. This article presents only a glimpse into a system likely to face physicians and patients in the foreseeable future.

Key Points

- Insurance is a mechanism to transfer risk.
- The price of that transfer depends, in large part, on the expected costs of services over the contract period.
- Expected use is determined, in part, by the experience of the group of insured.
- Claims data may be the only available source of experience data; however, analysts must recognize that use of services is driven by business practices and benefits levels.
- Insurance is a legally binding, aleatory contract; contributions from the insured and the insurer may not be equal.
- To "indemnify" is to reimburse for a loss; indemnity plans reimburse for expenses incurred.
- Insurers use medical underwriting to determine whether to accept a risk determined by medically relevant attributes of the insured.
- Reinsurance is used to transfer risk from an insurer to another insurer.
- Medicare's payment policies heavily influence private insurance policies and methods.

References

[1] Employee Benefit Research Institute Education and Research Fund. History of health insurance benefits. Washington, DC: Employee Benefit Research Institute; 2002.

[2] Stone DA. The struggle for the soul of health insurance. Journal of Health Politics, Policy and Law 1993;18(2)287–31.

[3] Andersen R. Revisiting the behavioral model and access to medical care: does it matter? J Health Soc Behav 1995;36:1–10.

[4] Andersen R, Newman JF. Societal and individual determinants of medical care utilization in the United States. Milbank Memorial Fund Quarterly 1973;51:95–124.

[5] Gabel J, Levitt L, Holve E, et al. Job-based health benefits in 2002: some important trends. Health Affairs 2002;21(5):143–51.

[6] Society of Actuaries. Principles underlying actuarial science. Exposure draft 1. Schaumberg (IL): Society of Actuaries; 1999.

[7] Brotman BA. Examining the existence of the underwriting cycle in managed care organizations. Journal of Health Care Finance 2000;27(1):50–4.

[8] Eisen, Roland. 1991. Problems of equilibria in insurance markets with asymmetric information. In: Henri Loubergé, editor. Risk, information and insurance: essays in the memory of Karl H. Borch. Boston: Kluwer Academic Publishers; 1991.

[9] Pauly MV, Nicholson S. Adverse consequences of adverse selection. Journal of Health Politics, Policy and Law 1999;24(5):921–30.

[10] Mehr RI, Cammack E. Principles of insurance. Homewood (IL): Richard D. Irwin; 1980.

[11] Taylor G. Loss reserving: an actuarial perspective. Boston: Kluwer Academic Publishers; 2000. p. 262–6.

[12] Schnieper R. On the estimation of the credibility factor: a Bayesian approach. Astin Bulletin 1995;25(2):137–51.

[13] The Lewin Group. Establishing an analytical framework for measuring the role of reinsurance in the health insurance market. Washington, DC: Department of Health and Human Services; 1997.

[14] Ellis RP, McGuire TG. Insurance principles and the design of prospective payment systems. Journal of Health Economics 1988;7:215–37.

[15] Keeler EB, Carter GM, Trude S. Insurance aspects of DRG outlier payments. Journal of Health Economics 1988;7:193–214.

[16] Schoenman JA, Hayes KJ, Cheng CM. Medicare physician payment changes: impact on physicians and beneficiaries. Health Affairs 2001;20(2):263–73.

[17] Iglehart JK. Medicare's declining payments to physicians. N Engl J Med 2002;346:1924–30.

[18] Health Committee of the Interim Health Standards Board of the American Academy of Actuaries. Actuarial Standard of Practice No. 5. Incurred health and disability claims. Rev. edition. Washington, DC: American Academy of Actuaries; December 2000.

[19] Fuchs VR. What's ahead for health insurance in the United States? N Engl J Med 2002;346(23):1822–4.

Address reprint requests to

Kyle L. Grazier
Department of Health Management and Policy
School of Public Health
109 South Observatory Street
University of Michigan
Ann Arbor, Michigan

e-mail: kgrazier@umich.edu

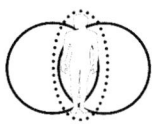
MAKING SENSE OF CODING FOR MEDICAL SERVICES

Eric Skye, MD, and Wendy Biggs, MD

The inception of Medicare in 1965 forever changed the face of American medicine. In conjunction, the American Medical Association (AMA) published the Current Procedural Terminology (CPT) in 1966, which listed the descriptive terms and identifying codes for reporting medical services and procedures performed by physicians. The CPT manual became the standard for billing codes. As an explosion of medical services provided to Medicare recipients occurred in the 1980s, the Health Care Financial Administration (HCFA), restructured as the Centers for Medicare and Medicaid Services (CMS) in 2001, sought to determine whether charges were submitted correctly. Because no documentation standards existed, the auditing of charts for accuracy of billing was dependent on the individual reviewer. The need for documentation guidelines to impart some consistency in assigning billing codes became apparent as medical record audits increasingly were used.

In 1994, HCFA, with assistance from the AMA CPT Advisory Panel, developed the first Documentation Guidelines (DGs). The DGs were implemented in 1995, and the medical community immediately called for revisions. The 1995 DGs provided a framework for documentation of evaluation and management (E/M) services, but disadvantaged physicians who examined only a single organ system. The DGs were revised and new guidelines were released for use in 1997. This newer system featured "bullets"—individual items in the PE that needed to be documented to receive "credit" for that organ system. This system was much easier for auditors, but frustrated many medical providers due to the counting of examination points it required. In response to the widespread criticism, the

From the Department of Family Medicine and Family Practice Residency, University of Michigan Medical School, Ann Arbor, Michigan (ES); and the Department of Family Practice, Michigan State University College of Human Medicine, Lansing, Michigan, and the Midland Family Practice Residency, Midland, Michigan (WB)

AMA CPT Advisory Panel and HCFA initiated yet another revision process. The AMA CPT Advisory Panel is currently in the process of revising the E/M codes. It is uncertain when newer revisions will become effective, although they currently are targeted for release in 2005. In the interim, physicians may use either the 1995 or 1997 DGs, "whichever is more advantageous for the physician."

This article discusses the 1995 and 1997 DGs for E/M codes. These guidelines are the original reference for the information contained in this article and are available at the CMS Web site [1]. We would like to issue the disclaimer that this article is for instruction, and is not meant to be the ultimate reference on coding. We recommend that you read the beginning pages of the most recent issue of the CPT manual [2], which outlines the accurate and up-to-date descriptions of codes for medical services and procedures. The CPT code set has been designated as the national coding standard by the Department of Health and Human Services and, as such, has been used as the reference for much of this article [2]. (The AMA's CPT manual can be obtained through the AMA press at 1-800-621-8335 or online at www.amapress.com.)

E/M CODING

Historically, family physicians have not always documented and therefore been given credit for the comprehensive nature of their office services. Office visits in a primary care office predominately are coded by using the CPT manual's section on "Evaluation and Management," and referring to the subsection on "Office or Other Outpatient Services" (99210–99215). Many family physicians assume that established patient visits should fall into a bell-shaped curve with the majority of visits being identified with the code 99213. However, family physicians often provide more comprehensive care then the simple problem-focused visits of the past. For example, in a practice with more complex or geriatric patients, the curve may be shifted more toward 99214 visits.

E/M coding is divided into three key elements: history, physical examination (PE), and medical decision making (MDM). Each of these elements, in turn, is divided further into components. The provider must consider each component to determine the level of the key element. The level of the three key elements then determines the E/M code of the office visit. This complexity has led many documentation tools to appear as grids, such as the one shown in Table 1.

History

The level of history is determined by four separate components: the chief complaint (CC); history of present illness (HPI); review of systems (ROS); and past medical, family, and social history (PFSH). To qualify for a given level of history, all four components must be considered (Table 2).

TABLE 1.
Evaluation and Management Coding Grid

	New Patients (Requires All Three Elements)					Established Patients (Requires Two of Three Elements)				
	99201	99202	99203	99204	99205	99211	99212	99213	99214	99215
History	PF	EPF	D	C	C	XX	PF	EPF	D	C
Examination	PF	EPF	D	C	C	XX	PF	EPF	D	C
MDM	SF	SF	LC	MC	HC	XX	SF	LC	MC	HC
Time	10 min	20 min	30 min	45 min	65 min	5 min	10 min	15 min	25 min	40 min

Abbreviations: C, comprehensive; D, detailed; EPF, expanded problem focused; HC, high complexity; LC, low complexity; MC, moderate complexity; MDM, medical decision making; PF, problem focused; SF, straight-forward; XX, not applicable.
Modified from University of Michigan Health System, Office of Professional Fee Billing Education and Compliance Monitoring Documentation Guidelines; with permission.

TABLE 2.
Determining the Level of History

History		Problem Focused	Expanded Problem Focused	Detailed	Comprehensive
History of present illness	Location	Brief (1–3)	Brief (1–3)	Extended >3	Extended >3
Descriptors	Severity				
	Timing				
	Quality				
OR	Duration				
	Associated signs				
	Context				
	Modifying factors				
Status of chronic or inactive diseases		0	1–2	3 or more	3 or more
Review of systems—14 systems	Constitutional	N/A	Problem pertinent 1	Extended 2–9	Complete
	Eyes				
	Ears, nose, throat, mouth				
	Cardiovascular				
	Respiratory				
	Gastrointestinal				
	Genitourinary				
	Musculoskeletal				
	Skin				
	Neurological				
	Psychiatric				
	Endocrine				
	Heme/lymphatic				
	Allergy/immunology				
Past medical, family, and social history		N/A	N/A	Pertinent 1 element	Complete >1 element

Abbreviation: NA, not applicable.
Modified from University of Michigan Health System, Office of Professional Fee Billing Education and Compliance Monitoring, Documentation Guidelines; with permission. *Data for modifications from* Centers for Medicare and Medicaid Services 1995 and 1997 Documentation Guidelines.

Each visit must have a CC; that is, why the patient is presenting to the clinician for evaluation. The clinician then elicits the description of the complaint from the patient. The recognized descriptors are location, quality, severity, duration, timing, context, modifying factors, and associated signs and symptoms. Alternatively, the status of chronic diseases can be mentioned within the HPI section. For example, "the patient's diabetes control is poor, with fingerstick blood glucoses in the 200s most days."

The next component of the history is the ROS. Fourteen systems are defined in the CPT manual, and the number of systems the provider addresses is the component that determines the level of visit. Pertinent negatives are acceptable; thus, if 10 systems are reviewed with the patient, the medical care provider can document the positive and select pertinent negative responses and then conclude, "a review of ten systems is otherwise negative." The final component of the history is the PFSH. The number of these elements addressed completes the level of the history.

The 1995 and 1997 DGs handle history similarly. For the health professional, the history often is the easiest component to determine in coding, and, frequently, the history is at a higher level of coding than the clinician expects. In optimizing coding, physicians should note that the difference in a problem focused (99212) and expanded problem focused (99213) history is as little as the review of one system. Most providers include some ROS in all histories, but may fail to recognize or document this. To meet the additional criteria for a detailed (99214) history, the HPI and ROS must be extended and at least one component of the PFSH needs to be reviewed. One of the most common coding errors is not taking credit for the detailed history that already has been taken.

PE

The PE component shows the greatest difference between the 1995 and 1997 DGs. Both systems recognize four different examination levels (problem focused, expanded problem focused, detailed, and comprehensive). The 1995 DGs use systems and body areas, whereas the 1997 DGs use a "bullet" system, in which the number of bullets completed determines the level of the PE. Clinicians should decide which system they are most comfortable with and consistently use that system. Either system involves counting to some extent. Table 3 provides a description of each body area and system along with the relevant "bullets." After determining the number of body areas or systems (1995 DGs) or the number of "bullets" (1997 DGs) that were examined, clinicians can determine the appropriate level of PE, as indicated in Table 4.

MDM

Assigning a level of complexity to the MDM element has been the most troublesome aspect of E/M coding. Three components comprise MDM: (1) the number of diagnoses or management options; (2) the amount or

TABLE 3.
Comparing 1995 and 1997 Physical Examination Guidelines

System or Body Area (1995 Guidelines)	Elements of Exam (Bullets) (1997 Guidelines)
Constitutional	☐Vital signs (at least 3)
	☐General appearance
Eyes	☐Conjunctiva and lids
	☐Pupils
	☐Fundoscopic exam
Ears, nose, mouth, and throat	☐External ears, nose
	☐Hearing
	☐Lips, teeth, and gums
	☐Nasal mucosa, septum, turbinates
	☐Oropharynx
	☐Otoscopic exam (canal and TM)
Neck	☐Neck ☐Thyroid
Respiratory	☐Effort ☐Palpation
	Percussion Auscultation
Cardiovascular	☐Auscultation of heart
	☐Palpation of heart
	Examination of:
	☐Carotid arteries
	☐Femoral arteries
	☐Abdominal aorta
	☐Extremities (edema, varicosities)
	☐Pedal pulses
Chest or breasts	☐Breasts (inspection)
	☐Breast and axilla (examination)
Gastrointestinal or abdomen	☐Exam of abdomen (mass, tender)
	☐Liver and spleen ☐Hernia
	☐Anus, perineum, and rectum
	☐Hemoccult test
Genito urinary	**Male**
	☐Prostrate exam ☐Genitalia
	Female
	☐External genitalia ☐Bladder
	☐Urethra ☐Cervix
	☐Uterus ☐Adnexa
Lymphatic/heme	Palpation in two or more areas:
	☐Neck ☐Groin
	☐Axilla ☐Other
Musculoskeletal	☐Gait and station
	☐Digits and nails
	Joints (one or more) (1) head and neck; (2) spine, ribs, and pelvis; (3) RUE; (4) LUE; (5) RLE; (6) LLE
	☐Inspection and palpation
	☐Range of motion ☐Stability
	☐Muscle strength/tone
Skin	☐Inspection ☐Palpation
Neurologic	☐Cranial nerves ☐Sensation
	☐Deep tendon reflexes
Psychiatric	☐Orientation ☐Mood and affect
	☐Recent and remote memory
	☐Judgment and insight

Abbreviations: LLE, left low ext; LUE, left up exx; RLE, right lower extremity; RUE, right upper extremity; TM, tympanic membrane.

Data from Centers for Medicare and Medicaid Services 1995 and 1997 Documentation Guidelines.

TABLE 4.
Comparison of Documentation Guidelines (DGs) for Physical Examination

	Problem Focused	Expanded Problem Focused	Detailed	Comprehensive
1995 DGs	1 Body area/system	2–7 Body area/ systems— limited exam	2–7 Body area/ systems— extended exam	≥8 Systems (not body areas)
1997 DGs	1–5 Bullets	6–11 Bullets	≥2 Bullets from six areas/systems or ≥12 Bullets from two or more areas/systems	≥2 Bullets from at least nine areas/systems

Data from Centers for Medicare and Medicaid Services 1995 and 1997 Documentation Guidelines.

complexity of medical records, diagnostic tests, or other information that must be obtained, reviewed, and analyzed; and (3) the risk of significant complications or morbidity or mortality. Four different levels of MDM are recognized—straightforward, low complexity, moderate complexity, or high complexity. Again, a gridlike approach is helpful in organizing this data (see bottom of Table 5).

MDM has proved difficult to formalize. A point system has been proposed by some to help determine the complexity of the MDM component (see Tables 5 and 6). Only two out of three elements are needed to determine the level of MDM. As an example of using the point system, moderate complexity MDM (99214) is achieved when a patient has a single new presenting problem or three established problems and a medication is prescribed. Analysis of other data or ordering other tests increases the MDM complexity. Many physicians undervalue their MDM, not realizing that many, if not most, office visits involve at least moderate-complexity MDM.

ASSIGNING E/M CODES

After the levels for the history, PE, and MDM are determined, these elements can be used to establish the level or billing code of the office visit. As noted in Table 1, a new patient, which is a patient not seen in that office for 3 years, must have all elements (three out of three) at the coded level. For an established patient, only two out of three elements are needed to bill at a given level. For example, even if the MDM is of moderate complexity and the clinician performs a detailed history and PE, the E/M code for a new patient would be 99203. For an established patient, the same history and physical would be coded as 99214, not 99213, regardless of the complexity of MDM, because only two components are required for established patients.

TABLE 5.
MDM Scoring System

Risk of Complications, Morbidity/ Mortality[a]	Number of Diagnoses and Management Options	Amount and Complexity of Data to be Reviewed	Level of MDM
	1 Point 1 Self-limited/minor problem 1 Established problem	1 Point Order and/or review clinical laboratory tests	
	2 Points 2 Self-limited/ minor problems	1 Point Order and/or review radiology tests except echo and cardiac catheter	
	2 Established problems 1 Established problem worsening	2 Points Direct visualization and independent review of image, specimen, or tracing	
	1 Stable chronic illness 3 Points	1 Point Discuss test result with performing physician	
	1 New problem— no additional workup planned 3 Established problems	1 Point Decision to obtain old records or history from someone other than the patient	
	2 Established problems, 1 worsening 4 Points	2 Points Review and summarize old records and obtain history from someone other than patient	
	1 New problem prob with additional workup planned 4 Established problems 2 Established problems worsening	2 Points Discuss care with other health care provider	
	— = Total points	— = Total points	

TABLE 5 *(continued)*

Risk of Complications, Morbidity/ Mortality[a]	Number of Diagnoses and Management Options	Amount and Complexity of Data to be Reviewed	Level of MDM
Minimal	1 Point—minimal	≤1 Point—minimal or none	Straightforward
Low	2 Points—limited	2 Points—limited	Low complexity
Moderate	3 Points—multiple	3 Points—moderate	Moderate complexity
High	4 Points—extensive	4+ Points—extensive	High complexity

[a] See Table 6.
Two out of three elements must be met or exceeded for a given level of decision making.
From the University of Michigan Health System, Office of Professional Fee Billing Education and Compliance Monitoring. Professional Fee Billing Guidelines for Teaching Physicians 1999; with permission.

Important for primary care providers is the provision that allows for billing based on time when counseling or coordination of care dominates the encounter (more than 50% of the actual visit time is spent on these activities). To assign a code based on time, the total length of time should be documented and the record should indicate what the counseling or coordination of care entailed. Common examples of counseling might include discussing diabetes and its care with a newly diagnosed diabetic, discussing lifestyle interventions with a patient, and so forth. The appropriate time intervals are indicated at the bottom of Table 1. The statement "greater than 50% of this XX minute visit was spent on counseling the patient regarding..." is a key phrase to remember when billing based only on time.

COMMON PITFALLS

Frequently, a provider is unable to bill for the level of work actually performed, due to inadequate documentation supporting the actual effort. Below are some common pitfalls and suggestions on how to avoid them:

1. Forgetting to document components of PFSH on an established patient on higher-level (99214 and 99215) visits.
   Suggestion: If you have a problem list that you keep updated, a remark of "PFSH updated on problem list" is sufficient. Commenting on these components within the body of your dictation also provides the needed documentation.
2. The ROS is not adequate.
   Suggestion: For a 99214, an extended ROS must include at least two systems. To document a complete ROS, pertinent negatives and positives must be recorded with a notation "all other systems

TABLE 6.
Risk of Complications

Level of Risk	Presenting Problem(s)	Diagnostic Procedure(s)	Management Options Selected
Minimal	Self-limited or minor problem	Laboratory test requiring venipuncture	Rest
Low	2 or more self-limited or minor problems	Superficial needle biopsies	Elastic bandages
	One stable chronic illness	Clinical laboratory test requiring arterial puncture	Superficial dressings
	Acute uncomplicated illness or injury	Single area roentgenograms	Over the counter drugs
		Physiologic tests without stress	Minor surgery with no identified risk factors
			Occupational therapy
Moderate	1 or more chronic illnesses with mild exacerbation	Physiologic tests under stress	Minor surgery with identified RFs
	2 or more stable chronic illnesses	Multiple area roentgenograms	Elective major surgery
	Acute illness with systemic symptoms	Deep-needle or incisional biopsy	Prescription drug management
	Acute complicated injury	Obtain fluid from body cavity	Closed treatment of fracture of dislocation without manipulation
	Undiagnosed new problem with uncertain prognosis	CT, MRI, bone scan	
		Cardiovascular imaging with contrast and no identified risk factors	
High	1 or more chronic illnesses with severe exacerbation	Discography	Elective major surgery with identified risk factors
	Acute or chronic illness or injuries that pose a threat to life or bodily function	Myelography	Emergency major surgery
	An abrupt change in neurologic status	Arthrogram	Parenteral controlled substances
			Drug therapy requiring intensive monitoring for toxicity
			Decision not to resuscitate or to de-escalate care because of poor prognosis

Abbreviation: RF,. Enter highest level of risk into first column of Table 5.

From the University of Michigan Health System, Office of Professional Fee Billing Education and Compliance Monitoring. Professional Free Billing Guidelines for Teaching Physicians 1999; with permission.

are negative," (If this phrase is not included, at least 10 systems must be documented individually.)

3. MDM does not appear to be of moderate or high complexity.

   Suggestion: Clearly state your clinical impression and differential diagnosis. Document your initiation of or changes in treatment. Record referrals to consultants. Include the tests ordered in the dictation. If a laboratory test or radiology test is reviewed, state this. Document decision to obtain old records. If old records are reviewed or additional history is obtained from the family or caregivers, a summary needs to be documented (saying "old records reviewed" is not sufficient). If you interpreted an electrocardiogram or roentgenogram, state so in the note.

4. The time recorded was not adequate for the level of the visit billed.

   Suggestion: Drill into your head "greater than 50% of this XX minute visit was spent on counseling the patient regarding..." and use it *every time* you bill, based on time spent counseling the patient.

5. The CC was not recorded.

   Suggestion: Every E/M visit must have a CC. Have your nurse or office staff record the CC. If you dictate, always start with "The patient presents with the complaint of X," and then proceed. (Preventive medicine visits do not require CCs.)

MODIFIERS

Modifiers are attached to E/M codes to explain to the insurance carrier when unusual or specific situations occur. Understanding and correctly using modifiers will ensure that your coding is accurate and you are getting credit for all of the work that you have performed. For a complete list of modifiers, please review Appendix A of the CPT manual.

Modifier 25 is the most common modifier code used in most primary care offices. When physicians provide "separately identifiable" services for a patient on the same day, they should submit both appropriate codes for the services and attach the modifier 25. The documentation must support each code reported. For example, you see a patient for follow-up of hypertension and note a skin lesion that you judge requires further management. The evaluation of this lesion would be incorporated appropriately into the office E/M code. If you took the time to treat this lesion with cryotherapy or remove it using a shave technique, you would add the appropriate procedural code and use the modifier 25 to indicate that this procedure, which was performed on the same day, was identifiably separate from the office visit.

PROLONGED SERVICES

The E/M codes for prolonged services (99354–99357) are available for use in conjunction with codes 99201 through 99215, 99241 through 99245, and 99301 through 99350 and are reimbursable, if the physician spends greater then 30 minutes of direct patient contact above and beyond the usual time for that service. As an example, usually you see a diabetic patient in the office for 25 minutes for review of blood sugars, diet, and exercise counseling and code a 99214 office visit. The patient is found to be hypoglycemic when his or her blood sugar is checked. You institute oral glucose and spend 1 hour of direct time with the patient. You would code this 99214 visit with the appropriate documentation, and also code a 99354 for the additional 35 minutes, making sure that you have described the nature of the prolonged service and the total time spent with the patient. These codes (with examples) are outlined clearly in the CPT manual.

PSYCHIATRIC PHARMACOLOGIC MANAGEMENT

Primary care providers often manage patients' anxiety and depressive disorders. Establishing patients' mental health diagnoses and initiating appropriate management are reported with E/M codes as discussed previously. For follow-up visits, if psychiatric diagnoses are one of several medical issues managed, it is appropriate to choose the proper E/M code. For follow-up visits involving *only* psychiatric medication follow-up, the proper code is not an E/M code but 90862. Physicians should evaluate and document the effect of the medication, any side effects, the dosage, and the interval in which they plan to re-evaluate the patient. The reimbursement of psychiatric codes has been problematic for many primary care providers because some insurance carriers may have specialty-specific policies regarding these codes. This is an area in which a discussion with intermediaries will help to anticipate their documentation and coding guidelines.

PREVENTIVE MEDICINE SERVICES

One of the most confusing areas in determining appropriate E/M coding is the delivery of preventive medical services. Prevention is considered a cornerstone of many primary care practices, yet variable reimbursement based on insurance carrier leads to differing interpreta-tions with regard to what is prevention and what is a medically necessary E/M service. The preventive medicine codes 99381 through 99397 are used for a periodic comprehensive preventive medical visit. The appropriate code is selected based on the patient's age and whether he or she is a new or established patient in the practice. Preventive medicine visits do not require a CC or a specific level of MDM to meet criteria; however, they do require the following components: an age-appropriate comprehensive history and physical, time spent in counseling, provision of anticipatory guidance, and discussion of care or behaviors targeted toward risk-factor reduction. The CPT guide states that the comprehensive nature of the history and PE for preventive services should be "age and gender appropriate" and may not be identical to the comprehensive history and physical defined for other E/M services.

The confusion occurs when these guidelines are applied to a real patient encounter, which is rarely a purely preventive visit. A patient visiting their physician for an "annual check up" often assumes that all of his or her chronic medical conditions will be reviewed and addressed, and also sees this visit as an opportunity to address other "minor" concerns. Some practices establish the expectation that only health-maintenance activities are addressed during an "annual physical." In general, if only "minor" or "insignificant" issues are addressed in conjunction with an annual examination that otherwise is intended to provide preventive services, then the visit should be coded as a preventive service, as described above.

If, however, a significant medical issue requiring further E/M presents during the preventive visit, and this medical problem is addressed, then the appropriate E/M office code (99201–99215) may be added to the preventive service code. The physician should indicate that this medical evaluation was a separately identified service, by attaching a modifier 25 to this service. For example, you are seeing Mrs. Jones, a 48-year-old smoker, for a preventive medicine visit that includes a Papanicolaou smear. Mrs. Jones is concerned about a cough that has worsened recently. You hear wheezing in her lungs during your PE and pursue other history to further evaluate the wheezing. You suspect she has chronic obstructive pulmonary disease with bronchospasm and order pulmonary function tests for further evaluation. You also prescribe an albuterol inhaler for her as initial management. In this case, you would be able to bill a 99213 with a modifier 25 in addition to coding Mrs. Jones's "annual check up" as 99396, because the visit was intended as a preventive services visit.

When identifying separate and significant E/M services during a preventive visit, the documentation must show the key components that were required above and beyond the preventive visit. Some practices advocate separate documentation for each visit code as a way to clearly identify to auditors the additional services performed, although this is not required by CMS. The reimbursement policy for two separate E/M services on the same day will vary by insurance carrier. Medicare allows both services to be reported; however, because preventive services are not a covered benefit, only the cost of the E/M office visit will be covered. A physician may not charge a Medicare beneficiary the complete cost of the preventive service visit in this situation, but must instead deduct the cost of the office visit and charge the beneficiary only the remaining balance. For example, you perform a periodic preventive examination (99397) and perform separate services supporting a 99213, which you have indicated with a modifier 25. If your office charges $150 for the preventive examination and $100 for the 99213 office visit, then you would bill Medicare for the $100 dollars and the patient would be responsible for the difference, or for $50.

Preventive medicine service codes also are available for individual counseling (99401–99404). These codes are used when an office visit is dedicated to individual counseling to promote health or prevention activities. The codes are based on time (15-minute intervals) and part of the documentation must include the total amount of time spent during this visit. If preventive counseling is provided on the same day that is separate from an E/M service, then a modifier 25 may be used to indicate these "separately identifiable services." For example, you see Mr. Jones for hypertension follow-up and he has questions about a planned trip to Central America. You spend an additional 15 minutes discussing prevention strategies during his planned travel. You would appropriately code the 99213 for his hypertension follow-up and add the 99401 with a modifier 25 to indicate this separate service.

PROCEDURES

It is crucial that primary care providers code procedures correctly. Procedures often are reimbursed at a higher level than are the E/M services in the office. If a procedure is performed during an office visit that has a separate E/M service (as is common with primary care providers), this should be indicated by assigning a modifier 25 to the procedure, indicating that it was separate from the E/M service. An example would be seeing a patient for a 6-month follow-up for diabetes, hyperlipidemia, and hypertension and assigning a 99214 for the E/M services associated with this visit. Then, the patient asks to have a wart frozen. If you perform the cryosurgery during the same visit, you should code it as a 17110 (destruction of lesion) and indicate with a modifier 25 that this procedure was separate from the E/M services.

Skin lesions may be removed by several distinct procedures. Destruction usually involves surface treatment of the lesion with liquid nitrogen, electrocautery, or chemical ablation. For example, the destruction of benign lesions such as warts, actinic keratosis, or seborrheic keratosis is coded with a 17000 for the first lesion and a 17003 for each additional lesion up to 14. The destruction of flat warts or molluscum contagiosum on the body, however, is coded as 17110 (up to 14 lesions). Removal of skin tags are coded separately with a 11200 used for the first 15 skin tags regardless of the method of their removal. If more than 15 are removed, 11201 is added for each additional 10 skin tags.

Removal of other skin lesions is coded properly by first assigning the correct size, location, and type of procedure. The two most common procedures for removing skin lesions include excision and shave techniques. Shaving is the sharp removal of a lesion without a full thickness excision and does not require closure. Shave procedures are reported using the codes 11300 through 11313, which include associated local anesthesia and any cauterization. Excisions are the complete full-thickness removal of a lesion and the associated simple closure of the wound (11400–11646). If the closure includes multiple tissue layers, then the appropriate intermediate (12031–12057) or complex closure (13100–

13153) codes should be included. Before 2003, these procedures were coded by the size of the lesion, not the excision. In 2003, however, this coding changed. The code for size now is determined by measuring the greatest diameter of the lesion plus the narrowest margins (ie, the shorter diameter of the ellipse or fusiform shape) made before excision (Fig. 1). Finally, the appropriate code and reimbursement is different depending on whether the lesion is determined to be benign or malignant on pathology, even if the procedure performed to remove the lesion is not different. Thus, many providers do not bill for these procedures until the final pathology is available to code the procedure correctly.

A biopsy is handled differently from an excision in coding. If a lesion is removed completely (even if this is done with a surgical "punch biopsy" instrument), it should be coded as an excision, as described above. If, however, a biopsy of a lesion (such as a punch of a portion of a lesion or rash) is performed for diagnostic reasons, then the code 11100 (biopsy of skin lesion) should be used. Biopsies are coded by the number performed and the code 11101 should be added for each additional biopsy performed.

Most minor surgical procedures are "bundled"—the anesthesia procedure, whether local or regional, and all the postoperative visits are included in the same code. If the wound becomes infected and the patient needs to be seen for additional visits, the office visits are included in the surgical code or "global fee." If a procedure was performed by someone outside of the practice, and the patient is seen afterward for care, the services are not included in the global fee, and the physician may bill for the appropriate E/M code.

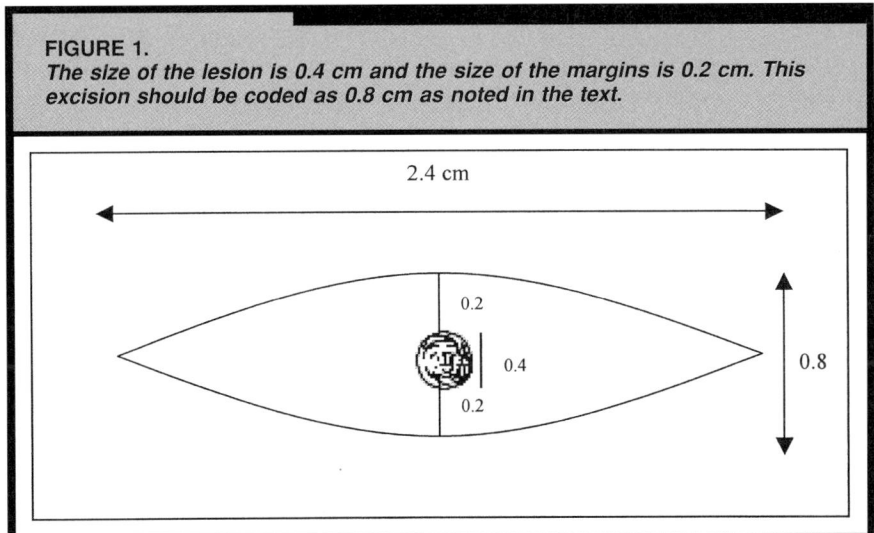

FIGURE 1.
The size of the lesion is 0.4 cm and the size of the margins is 0.2 cm. This excision should be coded as 0.8 cm as noted in the text.

Soft tissue injections and aspirations are common office-based procedures in a primary care practice. The codes for the aspiration or injection of a joint or bursa are the same, but differ with regard to the size of the joint. For instance, small joints (fingers, toes) are coded as 20600, intermediate joints (elbow, ankle) are coded as 20605, and large joints (knee, shoulder) are coded as 20610. A ganglion cyst aspiration or injection recently has been assigned a separate code and now should be reported as 20612. Coding of trigger point injections are determined by the number of muscles injected, with single or multiple trigger points in one or two muscles coded as 20552 and single or multiple trigger points in three or more muscles coded as 20553.

When providing care for musculoskeletal injuries that require casting or splinting, different codes exist depending on whether comprehensive management and follow-up or solely stabilization and transfer care to an orthopedist are provided. If a cast, strapping, or splint is applied to stabilize or protect an injury or fracture before transfer of care, the codes used are 29000 through 29580 (Application of Casts and Strapping). However, if the provider assumes all the subsequent care of a fracture and applies any appropriate splint or casts, then the codes in the 21000 through 28000 sections should be used instead. The application of necessary subsequent casts and splints then can be reported additionally using codes 29000 through 29850. If the provider applies a cast or brace, such as with an ankle sprain, and no other treatment or procedure is expected, this is properly reported with the appropriate E/M code (such as 99213) plus a supply code (99070) for the material or equipment used.

If certain procedures are performed routinely, it is important that physicians remember to read annually the CPT manual with regard to the proper billing of the procedures, because important changes can occur. For instance, in 2003, colposcopy coding was markedly revised. Instead of an inclusive fee, different codes now exist for each portion of the examination (such as examination of the cervix, vagina, and labia), with additional codes for biopsy and endocervical canal curettage.

HOSPITAL SERVICES

The principles of the E/M codes for inpatient hospital visits are similar to those for outpatient visits. The same three elements of the HPI, PE, and MDM are determined and then the level of the service is assigned. Initial hospital care requires all three elements to meet the coding level (as with a "new" outpatient visit), whereas subsequent care days require only two of the three elements (as with "established" visits). The initial hospital care visit applies to the first patient encounter by the attending physician and includes the admission history and physical. Although this occurs frequently on the day of admission, it is not uncommon for a patient to be admitted to the hospital in the evening and for the initial visit to occur the following day when the physician arrives at the hospital. In this situation, the initial visit, history, and physical would be billed on the day the patient actually was seen.

In contrast to the outpatient setting in which five E/M levels exist, there are only three levels for inpatient care. The lowest initial evaluation code (99221) requires a detailed history (HPI, four elements; ROS, two through nine systems; and PFSH, one element), and detailed PE (extended examination of two to seven systems or 12 "bullets"), but only straightforward or low-complexity MDM. The higher-level codes (99222 and 99223) require a comprehensive history and physical as well as moderate-complexity or high-complexity MDM, respectively. If the attending physician sees the patient in another setting (office, skilled nursing facility, or emergency department) before admission, all services provided by that physician should be combined to determine the initial code.

If a physician places a patient in the hospital for an observation period, the codes for inpatient observation (99234–99236) are used and determined similarly to initial inpatient days. If the patient subsequently needs to be admitted to the hospital during that 24-hour time frame, all service provided should be considered in determining the initial hospital evaluation code, which is the only code that should be submitted for the initial day.

Subsequent hospital days require at least two out of three elements to determine the level. Only three levels apply, and can be remembered as levels 1, 2, and 3: 99231, problem-focused/low-complexity MDM; 99232, expanded problem focused/moderate-complexity MDM; and 99233, detailed/high-complexity MDM, respectively. On the final day that the patient is in the hospital (the "discharge day" is reported separately based on the time the provider spends coordinating the discharge plans for the patient), either code 99238 (less than 30 minutes) or code 99239 (more than 30 minutes) is used. The time spent does not need to be conducted continuously, and includes preparing the discharge medications and documents and speaking to discharge planners, visiting nursing services, and family caregivers. If the time spent is more than 30 minutes, then the amount of time spent and a summary of actions should be included in the discharge summary.

It is important to bill for hospital care promptly. If multiple physicians are seeing a patient as "co-management" for subsequent hospital care, some insurance carriers will reimburse the first charge submitted and deny subsequent claims. Physicians should submit the bill with the diagnoses of the patient's medical problems that they are managing. If they are managing a patient for his or her medical problems after surgery, a formal consultation from the surgeon will enable them to bill for their services.

CONSULTATIONS

Consultations are important to differentiate from routine E/M visits, because documentation requirements and reimbursements are different.

Initial consultations can be performed in the hospital (codes 99251–99255) and the outpatient setting (codes 99241–99245), but the components to determine the level of the initial consult essentially are the same as in the E/M office visits (Table 1). Two features not required in routine E/M visits must be present in a consult: a request and a reply. For example, a physician or provider must request in writing your professional services regarding the E/M of a specific problem. In return, you must provide a written summary (consult) to the requesting provider. The problem that was evaluated and the provider who requested the consult should be documented clearly in the written consult note.

The most common pitfall in outpatient consultations for a family physician is the "preoperative consult." There is no code for "preoperative consult" or "clearing patient for surgery." The surgeon should make a request in writing with regard to the patient's medical problem(s) on which he or she would like the physician to render an opinion. Thus, the family physician would be doing a consultation. For example, "Dr. Jones requests that I see Mrs. Smith for evaluation of her diabetes and hypertension. She is scheduled for a carotid endarterectomy in 2 weeks." To complete the consult, you also must send a report to Dr. Jones outlining your evaluation and recommendations for Mrs. Smith's medical care before surgery.

After the initial consult, if the consultant initiates treatment and continues to participate in the patient's hospital care ("co-manage"), then subsequent hospital day codes should be used (99231–99233), not subsequent inpatient consultations. Subsequent inpatient consultation codes (99261–99263) are reserved for visits to complete only the initial consultation, such as follow-up of laboratory values or other tests when no further comanagement of the patient is expected. Another example occurs when the consultant completes a consultation and on another day is requested to see the patient again for exacerbation of the original medical problem. Subsequent inpatient consultation codes would be appropriate in this circumstance. If follow-up is performed in the outpatient setting, established patient office codes (99212–99215) should be used.

SUMMARY

Primary care providers are delivering increasingly complex care in today's health care system. With an understanding of the coding guidelines, physicians have the opportunity to clearly document and be reimbursed for the complex medical services that they provide. It is important that physicians avoid the common pitfalls of undercoding outpatient visits, not reporting separately identifiable services (modifier 25), and not taking credit for the time spent counseling patients. A clearer understanding of coding guidelines will allow physicians to streamline documentation, optimize coding, increase reimbursement, and minimize the likelihood of problems with auditors in the future.

Key Points

- One of the most common coding errors is not taking credit for the detailed history that has already been obtained.
- Many physicians undervalue their MDM, not realizing that many, if not most, office visits involve at least moderate-complexity MDM.
- A new patient, which is a patient not seen in that office for 3 years, must have all elements (three out of three) to bill at the coded level.
- An established patient requires only two out of three elements to bill at a given level.
- The statement "greater than 50% of this XX minute visit was spent on counseling the patient regarding..." is a key phrase to remember when billing based on time only.
- If a significant medical issue requiring further E/M presents during a preventive visit, and this medical problem is addressed, a physician may add the appropriate E/M office code (99201–99215) to the preventive service code.
- It is not uncommon for a patient to be admitted in the evening to the hospital and for the initial visit to occur the following day when the physician arrives at the hospital. In this situation, the initial visit, history, and physical would be billed on the day that the patient actually was seen.
- To bill for a consult, a physician or provider must request in writing another physician's professional services with regard to the E/M of a specific problem.

References

[1] Centers for Medicare and Medicaid Services. Documentation guidelines for evaluation and management services. Available at: http://cms.hhs.gov/medlearn/emdoc.asp. Accessed October 5, 2003.
[2] American Medical Association. Current procedural terminology 2002. Chicago: AMA Press; 2001.

Address reprint requests to

Eric Skye, MD
Clinical Assistant Professor
Department of Family Medicine
University of Michigan
L-2003 Women's, Box 0239
Ann Arbor, MI 48109.

e-mail: eskye@umich.edu

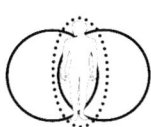
PROFESSIONAL AND PRACTICE MANAGEMENT SKILLS 1522–5720/03 $15.00 + .00

INTERPRETING PRACTICE FINANCIAL STATEMENTS

Quinta Vreede, MHSA

The financial aspect of any business often is one of the most difficult parts of that business to understand. This is clearly the case for many family practice clinics, in part because the physicians have not had any formal training in the field. This article introduces the three primary financial statements that are produced regularly: the balance sheet, income statement, and statement of cash flows. Mock financial statements are used to guide the reader through a practice analysis. This article, in addition to explaining the reports, also describes analytic tools such as ratios, key indicators, and forecasting; and discusses the benefits of comparison of actual performance to the previous period's performance, predicted performance (ie, budget), and benchmarks. The financial aspect of any business often is one of the most difficult parts of that business to understand. This clearly is the case for many family practice clinics, in part because the physicians have not had any formal training in the field. This article introduces the three primary financial statements that are regularly produced: the balance sheet, income statement, and statement of cash flows. In-house financial staff, an accountant, or a physician practice management company typically prepares the statements in accordance with the guidelines described in the Audits of Providers of Health Care Services (produced by the American Institute of Certified Public Accountants). This article describes a mock family practice and uses mock financial statements to guide the reader through a practice analysis. In addition to explaining the reports, the article also describes analytic tools such as ratios, key indicators, and forecasting; and discusses the benefits of comparison of actual performance to the previous period's performance, predicted performance (ie, budget), and benchmarks. By understanding these parameters, physician leaders will be better prepared to analyze decision-making events such as evaluating payer contracts, adding or removing a service, making versus buying decisions, and making

From the University of Michigan Hospital and Health Centers, Ambulatory Care Services, Ann Arbor, Michigan new equipment purchases. Additionally, physicians who are considering joining a practice will have a better understanding of how to evaluate the financial status of the practice.

SECTION ONE: FINANCIAL STATEMENTS

Accounting

Before discussing the actual financial statements, it is important to review what types of accounting systems can be used. Typically, small physician group practices use cash-based accounting systems. Cash-based accounting systems record the income or expense at the time the cash is either received or paid out. On the other hand, large practices or physician networks use accrual-based accounting. This type of accounting allows the practice to reflect projected income for the services already rendered as well as projected expenses.

The advantage to accrual-based accounting is that it can account for large revenue or expenses that are due to be received or paid. This minimizes the impact that large swings of cash generate and provides for more consistent reporting. Furthermore, it generally is required if the group needs to arrange for capital financing. One significant disadvantage to accrual-based accounting is that it records cash as if it were available but has not yet been collected, masking cash flow problems [1,2]. It also requires assumptions to be made with regard to what the payers will pay rather than what they actually do pay. Nevertheless, because accrual-based accounting is so widely used, for the purposes of this article, it is assumed that the mock family practice being discussed uses that system [1].

Balance Statement

A balance statement shows a practice's assets and liabilities. These two numbers must equal each other. Assets include three basic category groupings that represent either cash on hand, cash due (ie, accounts receivables), or items that have a monetary value (eg, inventories and equipment). Liabilities list amounts that are owed to another entity. Pending bills (accounts payable) and loans are examples of liabilities. The remainder is labeled equity. Assets and liabilities can be separated further into short-term and long-term categories that reflect the timing of the expected occurrence: short-term categories are for those items that will occur within a year [3].

Table 1 shows a balance statement for the mock family practice. In this table, the assets and liabilities added to the equity each equal $716,444 (lines 10 and 18) for the current year. Thus, as noted above, they must have the same value. The short-term assets include cash and investments, accounts receivable (adjusted for expected payment, ie, "net"), inventories, and other. These add up to $521,443 (line 6). The long-term assets

TABLE 1.
Balance Statement

		Current year
1	Assets	
2	Cash and investments	158,103
3	Accounts receivable (net)	314,925
4	Inventories	44,989
5	Other current assets	3427
6	Total current assets	521,444
7	Gross plant and equipment	257,775
8	Accumulated depreciation (less)	62,775
9	Total property plant and equipment	195,000
10	Total assets	716,444
11	Liabilities	
12	Accounts payable	195,074
13	Accrued expenses	31,448
14	Current portion of long-term debt	16,180
15	Total current liabilities	242,702
16	Long-term debt	149,500
17	Equity	324,242
18	Total liabilities and funds	716,444

include plant and equipment minus any dollars reserved to replace the asset (ie, depreciation) (line 9). As stated above the liabilities are divided into current liabilities (line 15, $242,702) and long-term debt (line 16, $149,500). The equity, also known as the net worth or fund balance, is $324,242 (line 17). A positive number means that the practice is making money [1].

Income Statement

The income statement also is known as a profit and loss statement and frequently is referred to by its abbreviation—P&L. This statement is broken down into three sections: income, expense, and margin (ie, the bottom line). Following along with the mock practice's income statement in Table 2 for the current year, the generated income is $2,347,020 (line 3) and the operating expenses total to $2,303,718 (line 19). This leaves income from operations (total revenue − total operating expense; line 20) of $43,302. Unlike the balance statement, which represents a point in time, the income statement reflects activity up to a given point in time—in this case, for the current year.

The income statement is the financial report that generates the most attention, because it provides a tremendous amount of information regarding both financial and operational measures and it gives the best look at the practice's profitability. In addition, it can be used to perform

TABLE 2.
Income Statement

		Current
	Operating revenue	
1	Net patient revenue	1,989,000
2	Other operating revenue	358,020
3	Total revenue	2,347,020
	Operating expenses	
4	Contracted services	29,900
5	Depreciation	26,140
6	Fringe benefits	217,251
7	Interest expense	11,960
8	Medical surgical supplies	95,000
9	Office supplies	45,858
10	Other	78,000
11	Payroll taxes	40,882
12	Professional liability	36,400
13	Promotion	8463
14	Rent	296,400
15	Equipment repair and maintenance	5340
16	Physician wages	801,125
17	Salaries and wages	561,600
18	Utilities	49,400
19	Total operating expenses	2,303,718
20	Income from operations	43,302
	Nonoperating gains or losses	
21	Contributions	—
22	Investment income	12,000
23	Total nonoperating gain	12,000
24	Excess of revenues over expenses	55,302

other types of analyses such as budgeting, trending, service analysis, and financial forecasting. Accordingly, a significant portion of this article will be devoted to examining the income statement in closer detail.

Income Statement: Income

The income section of the P&L refers to the revenue received for the services performed by the practice. It reflects all the services billed out at their expected reimbursement (if accrual based; otherwise, actual received payments if cash based) (see Table 2, line 1). The actual charges billed out to the patient or insurance company generally are reported in a billing summary report. Business units such as professional, laboratory, or testing revenue can be placed on a separate line (see Table 2, line 2).

One quick word with regard to gross charges, even though they are not presented formally on the income statement. In health care, physicians and payers enter into contracts, which determine the rate at which the physicians will be compensated for their services. Payers may set up contracts that pay at a straight percentage of charges, by fee schedule, or by capitation that uses a per member per month rate. These are recorded as contractual adjustments and can include bad debt. Net revenue (or income) is reported as gross charges net of any adjustments such as contractual allowances, and represents the cash received by the practice for the services provided. Looking again at Table 2, the total revenue for the practice is $2.347,020 (line 3). Insomuch as this mock practice is using an accrual-based accounting system, the contractual adjustments reflect assumptions regarding what will be received from the payers for the current billed services. A cash-based accounting system will reflect the cash received in that time period for previous services [1].

Income Statement: Expenses

Let's shift to the expense section of the income statement using the same example (see Table 2, lines 4–19). Expenses include all the payments a clinic has to pay out to produce the services generated at the practice. If the site is using cash-based accounting techniques, the income statements expenses reflect the dollars actually paid out by the practice. Accrual-based accounting, on the other hand, reflects the expenses incurred but not necessarily paid out [1]. The practice typically will categorize these expenses in what is called a chart of accounts. The accounts group similar expenses into categories to facilitate analysis and understanding. These typically include payroll, benefits, medical and surgical supplies, office supplies, insurance, rent, utilities, and depreciation. Moreover, expenses can be labeled as direct or indirect. Direct expenses are those expenses that can be tied to a specific service; for example, a syringe, office supplies, and pharmaceutical expenses can be tied directly to a particular vaccination. Indirect expenses are expenses that cannot be attributed to a particular billable event; for example, the cost of electricity or the cost of the office manager.

These expenses also can be described in terms of their relationship to activity levels and usually are referred to as fixed, variable, or semivariable expenses (Figure 1). By grouping these expenses in this manner, it is possible to facilitate the analysis of the income statement as is discussed later. Fixed expenses are those costs that a practice incurs regardless of the activity volume, and can include rent, housekeeping (typically paid on a square footage basis), and utilities. Variable expenses, on the other hand, reflect a category of costs that fluctuates proportionately with activity—for example, office and medical supplies. Finally, some expenses fall in between fixed and variable expenses, and sometimes are known as semivariable or step-variable expenses. These are expenses that change as volume changes but because they represent items that have capacity, it takes a large shift in volume to require an additional increment of expense [4]. A typical semivariable expense is payroll: a receptionist can handle up to a specific range of patients checking in before another receptionist is required.

When analyzing the expense section of the income statement, it is helpful to separate out the expenses by type. Fixed expenses, as stated

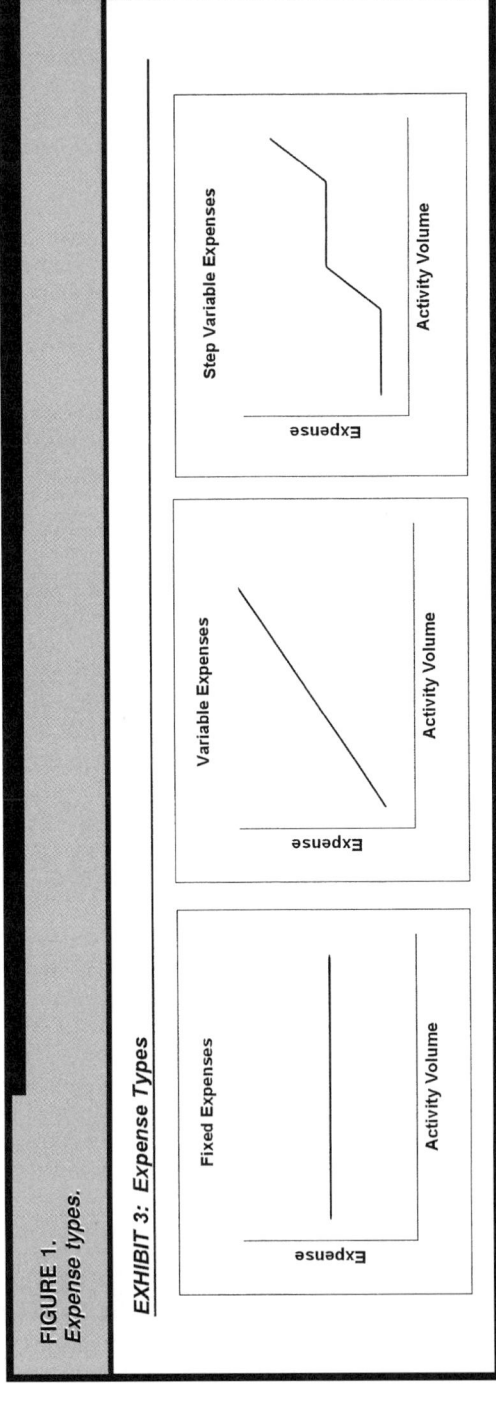

FIGURE 1.
Expense types.

before, are costs that are independent of volume. Thus, it is in the interest of the practice to ensure that these are "correctly sized" for the practice's activity, because as the volume goes up, the fixed expense per volume unit decreases. Keep in mind, however, that the best scenario may not be at the most extreme use—at some point diseconomies of scale set in. For example, too few examination rooms per physician can decrease the physician's productivity because the physician has to wait for the room to turn over. Therefore, strategies that use fixed assets effectively require significant correct sizing and balancing.

Variable expenses are viewed slightly differently. Because they are tied to volume, they are best looked at as part of a ratio with an activity unit as the denominator. By doing so, one can equalize for volume, which permits a better understanding of true unit cost. For example, with regard to office supply expense generated per visit, the more visits scheduled at the office, the more paperwork that is required.

Finally, semivariable expenses such as payroll have a particular relationship to a factor that contributes to changes in resource level. For example, medical assistants are most closely correlated with clinical physicians. Therefore, examinations of staffing levels generally show the support staff full-time equivalent (FTE) as a ratio to the physician FTE, regardless of the physician's productivity. Similar to fixed expenses, setting the optimal ratio is not necessarily the same as setting the smallest one.

Income Statement: Margin

Income from operations reflects what is remaining of the income after the operating expenses have been deducted. In the example in Table 2, the practice earned $43,302 from their operational activity (line 20). There also may be income from nonoperating revenue streams such as interest on investments or equity, and so forth. The addition of this type of income to the operational income produces a total margin that, for our mock practice, totals $55,302 (see Table 2, line 24).

Statement of Cash Flows

The presentation of the statement of cash flows typically is broken down into three sections to be of better use: cash flows from operations, cash flows from investing activities, and cash flows from financing activities. It also may include a fourth section titled cash flows from nonoperating. This statement describes the change in the cash holdings for the practice and generally is calculated by a combination of changes in the income statement and the balance statement [3].

For our mock practice, the statement of cash is presented in Table 3. The cash flows from operations ($53,695, line 1), investing activities ($7,733, line 2), financing activities ($7,459, line 3), and nonoperating cash flow ($12,000, line 4) indicate that there was a net increase of $50,503 (line 5) in cash for the practice's current year. This is added to the beginning

TABLE 3.
Statement of Cash Flows

Cash flow from operations	
Total operating revenue	2,347,020
Cash operating expenses	(2,277,578)
Change in accounts receivable	23,505
Change in inventory	6681
Change in other current assets	(227)
Change in accounts payable	(44,703)
Change in accruals	(1003)
1 Net cash flow from operations	53,695
Cash flow from investing activities	
2 Investment in plant and equipment	(7733)
Cash flow from financing activities	
3 Net cash flow from financing	(7459)
Nonoperating cash flow	
4 Nonoperating cash flow	12,000
5 Net increase (decrease) in cash	50,503
6 Beginning cash	107,600
7 Ending cash	158,103

cash, which is taken from the previous year's balance statement. The sum of these two numbers ($158,103, line 7) should equal the current year's balance statement (see Table 1, line 2).

SECTION 2: FINANCIAL RATIOS AND KEY INDICATORS

The three major financial statements can provide a vast amount of information to help physicians better understand the finances of their practice. This is accomplished partially through the use of ratios. The following discussion examines some key financial ratios and uses the financial statement examples to calculate and explore their significance.

Key Financial Ratios

- Operating margin
  Definition: Operating revenue less operating expense divided by operating revenue
  Data source: Income statement
  Example: (Table 2, line 3 – Table 2, line 19)/Table 2, line 3: ($2,347,020 – $2,303,718)/$2,347,020 = 1.84%
  Significance: Best gauge of the profitability of the practice; in other words, how much the practice makes for every operating dollar earned [3].

Related indicators: Total margin, which includes nonoperating gains (or losses) to examine how profitable the practice is when looking at all aspects of the business [3].

- Return on assets (ROA)
  Definition: Total revenue less total expenses, all divided by total assets
  Data source: Income statement and balance statement
  Example: (Table 2, line 3 – Table 2, line 19 + Table 2, line 23)/Table 1, line 10: ($2,347,020 − $2,303,718 + 12,000)/$716,444 = 7.72%
  Significance: This is also a profitability ratio calculating the dollars produced for each asset dollar. The higher the number, the more profitable the practice [3].

- Current ratio
  Definition: Current assets divided by current liabilities
  Data source: Balance statement
  Example: (Table 1, line 6)/(Table 1, line 15): $521,444/$242,702 = 2.15
  Significance: Calculates how much immediate cash is available relative to what is owed [3]. A ratio of 1.5 or greater is a good indicator of short-term liquidity [5].

- Days of cash on hand
  Definition: Cash divided by the difference between operating expense and depreciation expense divided by 365 days
  Data source: Balance and income statements
  Example: Table 1, line 6/(Table 2, line 19 − Table 2, line 5)/365): $158,103/($2,303,718 − $26,140)/365) = 25.34
  Significance: Indicates how many days the practice can cover its daily expenses if income ceases [3].

- Days in accounts receivable
  Definition: Total accounts receivable divided by average daily revenue
  Data source: Balance and income statements
  Example: Table 1, line 3/(Table 2, line 3/12): $314,925/($2,347,020/365) = 48.98
  Significance: Operational measure that reflects how well the accounts are being managed through the office billing functions. The higher the ratio, the longer it is taking to receive payment [5].
  Related indicators: Accounts receivable turnover, which uses 12 months instead of 365 days to derive average months [5].

- Debt ratio
  Definition: Total liabilities divided by total assets
  Data source: Balance statement
  Example: Table 1, line 15 + Table 1, line 16)/Table 1, line 10: ($242,702 + $149,500)/$716,443 = 55%

Significance: Used to determine the attractiveness to financing
institutions and the practice's ability to assume debt [3]. The
lower the number, the greater the ability to assume debt [5].

- Total asset turnover
  Definition: Total revenue divided by total assets
  Data Source: Balance and income statements
  Example: Table 2, line 3/Table 1, line 10: \$2,347,020/\$716,444 = 3.28
  Significance: Measures efficiency in how the assets are used. The
  higher the number, the more efficient the practice [3].
  Related indicators: Current-asset and fixed-asset turnover, which
  use current assets and fixed assets, respectively, instead of total
  assets.

The above indicators are summarized in Table 4, including benchmarks from the Medical Group Management Association (MGMA). The
practice is profitable, as determined by the operating margin and ROA. The
current ratio is consistent with similar practices and days of cash on hand
indicate that there is some cushion. The debt ratio and debt to equity
indicate that the practice has a lower than median debt and would be
considered a candidate for financing if needed. Because the practice rents
its facility and the debt position is relatively favorable, it should consider
modeling the benefits of a facility purchase.

Key Operational Indicators

The indicators reviewed below are derived primarily from the income
statement. It is common to see the income statement shown in comparison
with the results from the same period for the previous year (Table 5,
columns I and J) as well as in comparison with the current year's budget
(Table 5, columns E and F). Moreover, the report also may be produced to
include information for a given time period (generally a month or a quarter)
and for the performance for the year thus far (commonly referred to as
year to date or, in financial jargon, YTD). The indicators preferably should
be reported monthly, or at least quarterly, either by themselves or as part of
a management report that looks at all facets of the practice operations.

Income

Gross charges and net revenue should be trended over time. It is
important to keep in mind, however, that the fee schedule may have been
increased and the apparent increased income can be masking decreased
activity and future problems. It also is important to look at other indicators
that affect net revenue, physician productivity, billing process effectiveness, fee schedule, and payer contracts [2].

Physician productivity is measured best by using either net revenue
per physician FTE or work relative value unit (wRVU) per physician. Gross
charges per physician FTE is not a good measure for two reasons: (1)
physician practices have great latitude in establishing their price for

TABLE 4.
Key Financial Ratios

		MGMA Benchmark[a]	
	Current	Median	75th Percentile
Operating margin (%)	1.84	0.00	1.89
ROA (%)	7.72	0.00	9.38
Current ratio	2.15	2.13	4.55
Days cash	25.34		
Days in accounts receivable	48.98	45.55	56.66
Debt ratio (%)	55	69	85
Debt to equity	0.46	2.19	5.66
Total asset turnover	3.28	11.53	16.16

Exhibit Benchmark Sources: MGMA. Cost survey: 2002 report based on 2001 data.
MGMA. Physician Compensation and Production Survey: 2002 Report Based on 2001 data.
[a] *Data from* the Medical Group Management Association. Cost Survey: 2002 report based on 2001 data. Englewood (CO): Medical Group Management Association; 2002. Accounts Receivable Data, Collection Percentages and Financial Rations: Family

services, and (2) reimbursement contracts vary from place to place. Therefore, with gross margin, it is difficult to compare the practice against a national benchmark. Net revenue per physician FTE, on the other hand, is a better measure. However, this parameter can understate true productivity if there is an inefficient charge capture or billing process. The best indicator appears to be wRVUs per physician FTE. Not only is this a measure of the actual physician effort, but it also is easily benchmarked and is altered only by the effectiveness of the charge capture process (ie, how well the encounter forms are completed and billed).

To measure the billing process, the collection rate is one of the best starting points. Collection rate is defined as net revenue divided by gross charges. It measures how much of the services billed by the physician result in cash received. Thus, it is a reflection of the effectiveness of the billing services and insurance company contracts. Similar to gross charges, the collection rate is difficult to measure against a national benchmark because of the price self-selection [6]. Another indicator, net collection rate, measures how much cash is collected divided by how much cash should have been collected after adjusting for contractual allowances. After adjustments for bad debt, the target net collection rate for a practice should be in the mid- to upper 90% [7]. Other examples of billing drill-down indicators are days in accounts receivable, payer-specific collection rates, and rejection rates. This information is available from billing reports, and will give an indication of how clean the bills are (rejection rates), how promptly the payers pay (days in accounts receivable), and how well each payer is paying (payer-specific collection rates).

In Table 6, the practice's revenue and productivity indicators are calculated and compared with MGMA benchmarks. This comparison indicates that the wRVU/physician FTE is slightly below the median

TABLE 5.
Income Statement Variance Report

	A	B	C	D	E	F	G	H	I	J	K	L
	Current Month				Year to Date				Comparison to Previous Year to Date			
	Actual	Budget	Variance	% Variance	Current	Budget	Variance	% Variance	Actual	Previous	Variance	% Variance
Operating revenue												
1 Net patient revenue	165,750	186,567	(20,817)	-11.16	1,989,000	2,035,280	(46,280)	-2.27	1,989,000	1,976,000	13,000	0.66
2 Other operating revenue	29,835	31,409	(1574)	-5.01	358,020	342,638	15,382	4.49	358,020	335,920	22,100	6.58
3 Total revenue	195,585	217,976	(22,391)	-10.27	2,347,020	2,377,918	(30,898)	-1.30	2,347,020	2,311,920	35,100	1.52
Operating expenses												
4 Contracted services	2492	2323	(169)	-7.28	29,900	27,872	(2028)	-7.28	29,900	27,460	(2440)	-8.89
5 Depreciation	2178	2178	—	0.00	26,140	26,140	—	0.00	26,140	27,000	860	3.19
6 Fringe benefits	18,104	19,743	1639	8.30	217,251	215,383	(1868)	-0.87	217,251	208,566	(8686)	-4.16
7 Interest expense	997	997	—	0.00	11,960	11,960	—	0.00	11,960	12,275	315	2.57
8 Medical surgical supplies	7917	8947	1030	11.51	95,000	97,601	2600	2.66	95,000	94,300	(700)	-0.74
9 Office supplies	3821	4537	716	15.77	45,858	49,496	3639	7.35	45,858	48,765	2908	5.96
10 Other	6500	6833	333	4.88	78,000	82,000	4000	4.88	78,000	81,300	3300	4.06
11 Payroll taxes	3407	3719	312	8.39	40,882	40,567	(315)	-0.78	40,882	39,273	(1609)	-4.10
12 Professional liability	3033	3017	(17)	-0.55	36,400	36,200	(200)	-0.55	36,400	35,490	(910)	-2.56
13 Promotion	705	708	3	0.44	8463	8500	37	0.44	8463	2345	(6118)	-260.90

14	Rent	24,700	24,700	—	0.00	296,400	296,400	—	0.00	287,508	(8892)	-3.09
15	Equipment repair and maintenance	445	450	5	1.11	5340	5400	60	1.11	5320	(20)	-0.38
16	Physician wages	66,760	73,386	6625	9.03	801,125	800,573	(553)	-0.07	773,500	(27,625)	-3.57
17	Salaries and wages	46,800	50,570	3770	7.45	561,600	551,668	(9,932)	-1.80	535,600	(26,000)	-4.85
18	Utilities	4117	4032	(84)	-2.10	49,400	48,386	(1014)	-2.10	47,671	(1729)	-3.63
19	Total operating expenses	191,977	206,140	14,163	6.87	2,303,718	2,298,146	(5573)	-0.24	2,226,373	(77,346)	-3.47
20	Income from operations	3608	11,836	8228	69.51	43,302	79,773	36,471	45.72	85,547	42,246	49.38
21	Nonoperating gains or losses / Contributions											
22	Investment income	1000	973	(28)	-2.83	12,000	11,670	(330)	-2.83	11,300	(700)	-6.19
23	Total nonoperating gain	1000	973	(28)	-2.83	12,000	11,670	(330)	-2.83	11,300	(700)	-6.19
24	Excess of revenues over expenses	4608	12,809	8200	64.02	55,302	91,443	36,141	39.52	96,847	41,546	42.90

Current year budget assumptions: (1) Seasonality factor applied to revenue and variable accounts; (2) Fixed expenses allocated evenly across the months; and (3) Current year budget included the following adjustments from previous year's actuals; 1.5% increase for contracted services, office, equipment repairs, and utilities; depreciation, fringes, interest, and rent held constant; 3.5% increase for medical/surgical, physician salaries, and fringes; 3% increase for payroll and payroll taxes; and 2% increase in professional liability.

Exhibit Benchmark Sources: MGMA. Cost survey: 2002 report survey: 2002 report based on 2001 data. MGMA. Physician Compensation and Production Survey: 2002 Report Based on 2001 data.

TABLE 6.
Operational Indicators

	Year to Date				MGMA Benchmark	
	Current	Previous	Difference	% Change	Median	75th Percentile
Income						
Net revenue/physician FTE	361,080	355,680	5400	1.52%	436,454[a]	503,659[a]
Net income/physician FTE	6662	13,161	(6499)	−49.38%	—	8236[h]
wRVU/physician FTE	3850	3800	50	1.32%	3892[b]	4568[b]
Collection rate	79%	78%	0.80%	1.02%	69%[c]	77%[c]
Expense						
Visits per examination room per day	5.04	5.08	(0.05)	−0.94%		
Square footage per physician FTE	2000	2000	—	0.00%	1880[d]	2542[d]
PP&E expense per square footage	29.94	29.21	0.73	2.49%		
Building expense/net revenue	14.73%	14.50%	0.23%	1.61%	5.85%[e]	7.85%[e]
Equipment expense/net revenue	1.85%	1.83%	0.02%	1.18%	1.13%[e]	1.67%[e]
Medical surgical supplies/visit	3.42	3.48	(0.06)	−1.75%		
Office supplies/visit	1.65	1.76	(0.11)	−6.48%		
Medical surgical supplies/net revenue	4.05%	4.08%	−0.03%	−0.76%	4.18%[e]	4.78%[e]
Office supplies/net revenue	1.95%	2.11%	−0.16%	−7.37%	2.18%[e]	2.66%[e]
Support staff payroll/net revenue	29.0%	28.0%	0.92%	3.29%	31.26%[e]	37.54%[e]
Physician compensation/physician FTE	145,435	140,420	5,015	3.57%	146601[f]	180589[f]
Malpractice/physician FTE	5600	5460	140	2.56%	5419[g]	8840[g]
Total operating expenses per net revenue (not including physician compensation)	57.9%	56.8%	1.06%	1.86%	59.43%[e]	63.65%[e]

Skill mix breakdown (in FTEs) per physician						
FTE						
Business staff	2.50	2.60	(0)	−3.85%		
Clinical support staff	1.10	1.10	—	0.00%		
Nursing	0.50	0.50	—	0.00%		
Total	4.10	4.20	(0)	−2.38%	4.41[d]	5.62[d]
Operational statistics						
Gross charges	2,970,911	2,956,419				
Physician FTEs	6.5	6.5				
wRVUs	25,025	24,700				
Visits	27,806	28,068				
Square footage	13,000	13,000				
Examination rooms	24	24				

[a] Medical Group Management Association (MGMA) Cost Survey 2002 Report based on 2001 Data Table 10.4B Family Medicine Not Hospital Owned.
[b] MGMA Physician Compensation and Productivity Survey: 2002 Report Based on 2001 Data; Table 59.
[c] Medical Group Management Association (MGMA) Cost Survey 2002 Report based on 2001 Data Table 9.2 Family Medicine Not Hospital Owned.
[d] Medical Group Management Association (MGMA) Cost Survey 2002 Report based on 2001 Data Table 9.4a Family Medicine Not Hospital Owned.
[e] Medical Group Management Association (MGMA) Cost Survey 2002 Report based on 2001 Data Table 9.5b Family Medicine Not Hospital Owned.
[f] MGMA Physician Compensation and Productivity Survey: 2002 Report Based on 2001 Data; Table 1 Family Medicine (w/out) OB.
[g] Medical Group Management Association (MGMA) Cost Survey 2002 Report based on 2001 Data Table 9.4c Family Medicine Not Hospital Owned.
[h] Medical Group Management Association (MGMA) Cost Survey 2002 Report based on 2001 Data Table 9.4e Family Medicine Not Hospital Owned.

benchmark and has improved 1.32% over the previous year. Net revenue/physician FTE, also low when compared with a benchmark, improved even more over the past year, most likely due to an improved billing process, because the collection rate also improved by 0.8%. The collection rate when compared with the MGMA benchmark appears to be better than the median benchmark. This could be due to more favorable payer contracts, a better billing process, or a lower price schedule.

Expenses

Analysis of expenses should focus on the more expensive items, prepared as ratios, trended over time, and compared with benchmarks [8]. Expenses can be divided further into fixed and variable categories. The correction strategies for each of these vary, as discussed earlier.

Fixed Expenses. The following statistics should be looked at for fixed expenses:

- Visits per examination room (examination turnover rate): This statistic gives an indication of how well the examination rooms are being used in the practice. Keep in mind, however, that this is not adjusted for type of visit. In addition, good benchmarks are not available. Instead, it may be a good idea to look at this indicator and trend it over time.
- Square footage per physician FTE: This indicator gives a value as to how much space is allocated on a physician basis as compared with examination turnover rate, which measures how well examination rooms are being used, but does not address the space allocation between nonexamination and examination rooms. One point to keep in mind is how square footage is defined when comparing with benchmarks.
- Plant, property, and equipment (PP&E) expense as a percentage of net revenue: The PP&E gives an idea as to how expensive it is to maintain the facility. For comparative purposes, this statistic can be reduced to building as a percentage of net revenue and equipment as a percentage of net revenue. This type of analysis can be extended to all fixed expenses and compared with national benchmarks. Remember that improved productivity will reduce the cost per net revenue, even though the practice has not reduced its expenses.

Using the example practice statements along with some additional operating statistics, it is possible to derive these indicators as shown in Table 6. The examination room turnover indicates that the practice is averaging 5.0 visits per examination room per day. From a commonsense perspective, this appears to be relatively low, but could be affected by the complexity of the patients and the other obligations of the physicians (eg, covering inpatient calls or outpatient services at other locations). The square footage per physician FTE appears to be relatively high in comparison with other similar practices. This would indicate that there might be opportunity to use some of the extra space for additional revenue-generating activities by either bringing in another physician or service. The building and equipment expense as a percentage of net revenue also is high when compared with the MGMA benchmark. As the net revenue per physician FTE improves, this expense will decrease. However, this result also would indicate that the practice has an opportunity to either add a service to reduce the excess capacity, or—because the debt ratio is below the median and the rental rate is rather high—to consider purchasing a more appropriately sized building.

Variable Expenses. For variable expenses, it is best to look at the expense per unit of activity. The numerator can be any of the variable expenses such as medical or office supplies. The denominator generally is one of three items. Visits work well because variable expenses typically are incurred regardless of the patient's acuity; however, they are hard to benchmark externally because a visit can be hard to define. They are useful, however, in determining the cost of current services and projecting future growth or additional services. A second activity unit, wRVUs, also can be used as a denominator; however the variable supplies may not vary proportionally to the denominator changes, and this item cannot capture billable activity that does not have an assigned wRVU. A good indicator to compare with MGMA benchmarks is expense as a percentage of net revenue. Analysis of the practice's performance for medical, surgical, and office supplies indicates that the practice reduced these variable expenses on a unit cost basis from the previous year. A comparison with the benchmark indicates that the practice is efficient as well.

Semivariable Expenses (Payroll). Payroll should be analyzed either as a percentage of net revenue or as a ratio of support staff FTEs to clinical physician FTEs. Support staff FTEs:clinical physician FTEs is an important starting point in determining whether there is enough staff to support the clinic activity efficiently. The ratio of support staff FTEs to Clinical Physician FTEs can be broken down by types of employees as well (eg, office assistant, nurses, and so forth.). Examining payroll as a percentage of net revenue makes it possible to analyze how much it costs to produce that net revenue, which helps to examine the skill mix as well, because certain skilled employees cost more. Both of these indicators will assist in the determination of whether the skill mix is appropriate. One important point to keep in mind is that it is crucial for the practice to be staffed appropriately. Practices that either are overstaffed or understaffed can create financial problems—the former, by increasing costs and the latter, because physician time is not used appropriately (ie, physicians would need to perform tasks that should be done by others) [2].

Again, using the practice example financial statements, it appears that the support staff per physician FTE is a little low compared with the benchmark. Note that the MGMA individual benchmarks for the skill mix breakdown are not added because the medians are not additive and not all survey respondents employ the same labor types. Examining payroll as a percentage of net revenue also indicates that the support staff payroll is below the median benchmark. Coupling that statistic with the physician productivity at the median level may indicate that there is an opportunity to add staff to enhance the physician productivity. As stated previously, the examination room turnover rate appeared to be relatively low as well: improved physician productivity would improve the turnover rate. Of course, to further examine the viability of this project, the practice would need to develop a solid plan for how the incremental staff would be used to improve the physician productivity. Furthermore, the plan should determine how many more wRVUs would need to be generated to cover the incremental staff costs. Another important cost statistic, physician salaries (including fringe benefits), compares favorably with the MGMA benchmark. Support staff and physician payroll expenses for the practice account for just under 70% of net revenue. This statistic can be improved by productivity improvements up to a certain level, before staff needs to be added incrementally.

Other Expenses. Malpractice expense typically is looked at by physician FTE. As the FTEs grow, so does the malpractice expense. Malpractice per physician FTE or individual physician will permit the practice to compare their expenses against national benchmarks. The example's liability expense per physician FTE is a little bit higher when compared with the MGMA family practice median benchmarks.

Lastly, it is important to look at total expense as a percentage of net revenue (not including physician compensation). In Table 6, the practice's operating costs are consistent with national benchmarks and are trending consistent with inflationary increases. However, as noted in the preceding discussion, although things may look fine in the aggregate, there still may be opportunities to improve income and expense and net revenue by investing in some variable expenses.

SECTION 3: OTHER USES OF FINANCIAL STATEMENTS

Budgeting

In addition to preparing income statements, which reflect actual performance, many practices also use the income statement to project what they believe the coming year will look like. These are called either pro forma or budgets. Budgeting the P&L is important because it provides the road map for the performance expectations in the upcoming year. In addition, it identifies up front what some of the issues or barriers may be, thus providing an opportunity for practices to implement proactive remedies.

Budget Preparation

Budgeting can be presented in several ways. Most typically, a budget is prepared for the entire year, although there are many practices that do not do this, but adjust their operations as appropriate. Others prepare what is called a rolling budget— a budget that is prepared a few months at a time so as to have relatively updated numbers. An advantage of this approach is that it reflects a more current view of reality. Sometimes budgets are fixed (no changes permitted once the budget has been approved) and sometimes they flex with volume changes (ie, as volume increases or decreases, variable expenses increase or decrease). Regardless of the type of budget used, there always should be a year's view of expected performance.

There are several ways to start the budget preparation process. One way is to create a "zero-based" budget that starts with a fresh page and determines realistic numbers for the upcoming year. The MGMA's report, *Performances and Practices of Successful Medical Groups*, indicates that the better performing medical groups use the "zero-based" approach [9]. Others start with what they budgeted for the current year and then adjust for actual performance. Once the base is completed, then known changes for the following year or time frame are added and documented. In addition to these known changes, there are assumptions of what may occur in the future. These assumptions are documented as a footnote to the budget so that they are easily recognized and understood when examining the projected budget.

Budget Analyses

Because future assumptions often are a "best guess," it is helpful to conduct scenarios analyses that demonstrate the various assumptions and the effects that they would have on the practice's financial health. This can be accomplished by using a spreadsheet computer system such as Microsoft Excel. In addition to scenario analyses, there also are sensitivity analyses that gauge the effects of assumptions through a variety of values. Finally, it also is beneficial to determine a "break-even" point—the exact point at which the practice hits its targets, such as a 5% operating margin or dollar target.

Once the budget has been approved, it is then "calendarized." A time period is chosen that typically represents a month. The budget then is divided into 12 months, but also can be adjusted for seasonality. Seasonality is the concept that practices often vary throughout the year on a predictable basis. This is best determined by going back several years to identify historic performance and trends that are anticipated to be replicable in the future. When doing this, it is important to be aware of major changes on a practice mid-year that can give an appearance of seasonality (eg, adding a mid-level provider, having a physician off for an extended period of time).

Reporting Actual to Budget Performance

Once the budget has been developed and accepted, the financial statements should be updated for each month, comparing actual performance to budget. Table 5 models this for the mock practice. It also is helpful to show current performance against last year's performance for the same time period. Also reported are variances of actual performance from budget in terms of dollars and percentages. Percentages make it possible to identify quickly those items that have the greatest variance.

However, it is also necessary to look closely at actual dollars because each line item is not weighted equally. A better return on time investment can be obtained by explaining an unfavorable 4% variance in medical surgical supplies that represents $25,000 in increased expenses rather than a 35% expense variance that represents $1000.

Analysis of Table 5 shows that revenue for the mock practice has improved over the previous year's performance (1.52%, line 3, column L), but not as much as originally projected (-1.3%, line 3, column H). The expenses have increased over last year's expenses and the current year's budget (line 19, columns L and H, respectively). Much of the expense increase over last year was due to the planned salary increases for support staff (line 17, column K), physicians (line 16, column K), and fringe benefits (line 6, column K). Contractual rent increases along with the enhanced advertising expenses account for the remaining expense increases over the past year. Due primarily to the lower than expected revenue, the practice did not meet their margin expectations, even though they had a profitable year.

Forecasting/Trending

Financial statements, in addition to charting future performance expectations and monitoring actual performance, also can be a tool for analyzing historic trends to predict what will happen in the future if the trends continue. This important exercise feeds into the budget process. In addition to trending the statements, it is important also to trend the key indicators that were discussed earlier (Table 6). This will inform the practice of potential trouble spots ahead.

ADDING A SERVICE

A previous part of this article discussed whether adding a mid-level provider or another service to the practice would allow it to better use its fixed assets or whether adding a medical assistant would result in improved physician productivity. A financial analysis can be conducted that would allow for the forecasting of expected revenues (using benchmarks as a proxy). The variable expenses then would be incremented by the expected activity volume and current variable expense/activity volume indicators, while holding fixed expenses constant. This type of modeling makes it possible to identify quickly whether adding the service would result in a financial benefit and at what activity level the practice would break even on the investment. Indicators used to determine project viability can include return on investment or net present value. Important considerations not taken into account by this type of analysis are other services that may offer a higher return or better qualitative considerations, such as improved patient satisfaction, better access, and so forth.

EXAMPLE SUMMARY

The mock family practice example can be summarized in the following way. The practice is profitable with some ability to handle debt. It appears to have a good billing process approach and is able to keep its expenses in line. Most of the practice's profitability stems from the tight control over expenses and business processes. Opportunities for the clinic based on the analysis of the financial statements indicate that the facility costs appear to be high and the physician productivity could be improved. These factors might be able to be improved by the purchase of an appropriate-sized building and the careful addition of support staff to enhance clinical operations and physician productivity.

SUMMARY

Although the practice with which a person is affiliated may present its financial information differently than the one presented in this article, the concepts should be replicable. The key is to look at the statements and calculate the ratios and indicators on a regular basis. Trending of this information and comparing it to benchmarks will facilitate quick iden-tification of potential trouble spots. Furthermore, ratios and indicators can provide valuable input with regard to determining whether services will be of financial value to the practice.

Key Points

- The three primary financial statements that form the foundation for any financial analysis are the Balance Statement, Income Statement and Statement of Cash Flows.
- Calculation of a few financial ratios will provide the necessary data to examine a practice's current financial health
- Key operational indicators will shed light on how efficiently the practice is operating and can identify targeted areas for improvement
- Projections and scenarios of the income statement will provide an important look at the practice's future direction.
- A solid understanding of the practice's financial and operational indicators will permit better decision-making for business situations such as evaluating payer contracts, adding or removing a service, and making a new equipment purchases.

References

[1] Preston S. Accrual accounting: easy as 1,2,3. Medical Economics 1998;June 29:75–80.
[2] Halley MD, Little AW. Net one, net two: the primary care network income statement. Healthcare Financial Management 1999;53(10):61–3.

[3] Gapenski L. Financial and operating analysis. In: Understanding health care financial management: text, cases and models. Ann Arbor (MI): AUPHA Press/Health Administration Press; 1993; p. 539–93.

[4] Tipton EF, Finley JB. The "fixed cost effect" on practice management. MGM Journal 1999;July–August:28–31.

[5] Schryver DL. Financial ratios and group practice operations. MGM Journal 2000; September–October:14.

[6] Fry C. Developing a corrective-action plan for the revenue cycle. Healthc Financ Manage 2001;55(5):61–6.

[7] Tuttle G. A simple way to monitor your practice's vital signs. Medical Economics 1996;March 11:135–45.

[8] Wood KM, Matthews GE. Reviewing practices expenses can improve profitability. Healthc Financ Manage 1997;51(7):81–3.

[9] Jaklevic M. Practices with the best practices: with many doc groups losing money, MGMA study shows what makes a "better performer." Modern Healthcare 1999;February 8:64–5.

Address reprint requests to

Quinta Vreede, MHSA
University of Michigan Hospital
Ambulatory Care Services
7300 Dexter Ann Arbor Road
Box 0474
Dexter, MI 48130

e-mail: qvreede@med.umich.edu

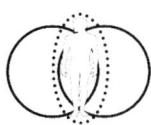

PROFESSIONAL AND PRACTICE MANAGEMENT SKILLS 1522–5720/03 $15.00 + .00

PHYSICIAN PRODUCTIVITY AND REIMBURSEMENT

Jean M. Malouin, MD, MPH

Whether you have been in practice many years or are a recent residency graduate, it is likely that productivity and reimbursement issues are now an unavoidable and perhaps unwelcome part of your professional life. Physician reimbursement mechanisms have undergone dramatic changes over the past 10 years and some of these changes have significantly altered the way in which family physicians provide care for their patients. It is no longer enough to simply provide quality medical care; it must now be done while maximizing efficiency and cost effectiveness. If this does not happen, then incomes will suffer. Understanding what is expected of physicians and how they will be reimbursed for the work they do is more important than ever.

This article describes common methods for measuring physician productivity and defines how these productivity measures may be used as part of a compensation plan for reimbursing employed physicians. It is intended for use as a resource for physicians who are responsible for designing and implementing salary programs and to help physicians understand their own personal income potential and compensation plan.

PHYSICIAN PRODUCTIVITY

Defining Physician Productivity

Physician productivity is a measure of a physician's work or output. It can be expressed in various units including patient visits, gross charges, or net charges. One common method for defining physician productivity is the relative value unit (RVU). This unit is defined by the Resource-Based

---

From the Department of Family Medicine, University of Michigan Medical School, Ann Arbor, Michigan

Relative Value Scale, introduced by the Health Care Financing Administration (HCFA) in 1992 for Medicare reimbursement and now adopted by many other third-party payers. According to the American Medical Group Association's 2001 Medical Group Compensation and Productivity Survey, the percentage of medical groups reporting that they used RVUs as a measure of physician productivity rose from 8% in 1999 to 28% in 2000 [1] and continues to rise. There is a gradually increasing awareness of the value of using RVUs to measure productivity, probably because this system accounts for the complexity and intensity of care in a manner that cannot be quantified accurately by using visits or gross revenue as productivity markers. Because of this trend, the focus of this article is primarily on RVU-based reimbursement mechanisms.

The RVU system used for reimbursement by the Centers for Medicare and Medicaid Services (CMS) includes a physician work component, a practice expense component, and a malpractice cost component. The work component accounts for approximately 55% of the total RVU value, whereas practice expenses and malpractice costs account for approximately 41% and 4%, respectively [2]. In general, the physician work component is what is used to track physician productivity. It assigns a numeric value to each Current Procedural Terminology code that is designed to quantify, in relative terms, the amount of work that a physician performs for each type of service. Table 1 lists work RVU values for several common physician services [2].

However, RVU measurements alone do not tell the whole tale with regard to physician productivity. It also is important to measure efficiency, which can be thought of as productivity in a measured time period (for example, visits per hour). This is a more accurate way to quantify productivity, because it takes into consideration the resources needed to

TABLE 1.
Comparison of RVUs for Select Physician Services

Service	CPT Code	Work RVUs
Office visit, detailed, established patient	99213	0.67
Colposcopy with biopsy	57454	1.27
Excision of benign skin lesion	11401	1.32
Office visit, detailed, new patient	99203	1.34
Office visit, complex, established patient	99215	1.74
Inpatient consultation	99254	2.64
Initial hospital care	99223	2.99
Routine prenatal care and delivery	59400	23.06

Abbreviations: CPT, Current Procedural Terminology; RVU, relative value unit.

produce the output. A physician who sees 15 patients in a 4-hour period is more efficient than one who sees the same 15 patients in an 8-hour period.

Setting Productivity Benchmarks

Most organizations that measure and monitor physician productivity also set target or "benchmark" productivity levels. These benchmarks may be set based on internal practice performance standards, such as the 75th percentile of annual productivity in the group. Alternatively, many practices use external data published by the Medical Group Management Association (MGMA). This organization regularly publishes data on physician productivity and compensation, and defines benchmarks for staffing per physician full-time equivalent (FTE).

Productivity benchmarks may be based on total annual RVUs, RVUs per hour, or RVUs per session. MGMA reports mean, median, 25th percentile, and 75th percentile values for annual RVUs by specialty. The MGMA 2002 Physician Compensation and Production Survey annual work RVUs for family practice physicians are summarized in Table 2 [3]. The data are based on full-time employment status and, therefore, these numbers must be adjusted for part-time or academic-based physicians with nonclinical responsibilities.

It is important that the goals being set are reasonable and at least conceptually achievable. If a practice is required to operate with less than optimal staffing and there is little chance that this will change, it may not be reasonable to hold physicians accountable for meeting benchmark productivity levels that were achieved using greater resources.

Accounting for Capitation

Many practices have a high percentage of managed care patients for whom they are reimbursed by a capitated method. This means that the physician is paid a fixed per-member-per-month rate for each enrolled patient. The practice gets the same reimbursement whether the patient is seen weekly or not at all. Obviously, under this model an incentive system

TABLE 2.
Annual Physician Work Relative Value Unit for Private Practice Physicians

	Mean	25th %ile	Median	75th %ile
Family practice with obstetrics	4361	3435	4169	5177
Family practice without obstetrics	3980	3221	3892	4568

that rewards productivity based on visits or RVUs generated is a system that is not strategically aligned with payer reimbursement. In purely capitated systems, financial gain is maximized by keeping the patient out of the clinic. The ethical and quality issues that this may raise are beyond the scope of this text; however, it must be pointed out that a system that rewards productivity under capitation is a system that may be missing the point financially. Practices that derive a large percentage of their income from capitated revenue are more likely to base physician compensation on measures of quality and use rather than physician productivity [4].

Many clinics have a blended mix of capitated and fee-for-service patients. Based on information from the CMS, approximately 91% of physicians have at least some percentage of managed care patient enrollment. Of this managed care enrollment, 63% are reimbursed using a capitated method [5]. Under this blended model, it may make sense to have an incentive system that rewards physicians based on a weighted mix of productivity, patient panel size (number of patients signed up with a particular provider), and quality measures such as Health Employer Data Information Set (HEDIS) measures and patient satisfaction.

Factors Influencing Physician Productivity

There are many variables that influence physician productivity, although their relative weights tend to differ from person to person. Whether you are an individual physician trying to increase your own productivity or a medical director trying to influence your group's productivity, a thorough understanding of the factors contributing to productivity levels is important. These factors are as follows: (1) knowledge of coding and billing, (2) physician practice style, (3) part-time or full-time employment status, (4) scope of practice, (5) patient case mix and complexity of care, and (6) office efficiency.

Knowledge of Coding and Billing

Reimbursement from third-party payers is highly dependent on accurate coding and billing. Two physicians can both see three patients per hour and provide the same level of care; however if one of them is "coding savvy" and one is not, their reimbursement may be dramatically different. Family physicians often feel that they are undervalued by the health care system and undercompensated for their work, yet tend to have some resistance to learning coding behaviors that will legally allow them to be adequately reimbursed for their efforts. Some of this resistance is due to the fear that they will inadvertently overbill and be accused of Medicare fraud; however, some likely is due to the resistance to change that is inherent in human nature. Whatever the reason for undercoding, physicians need to understand that they can and should be reimbursed to the maximal allowable level for the services they perform. According to the American

Academy of Family Physicians (AAFP) 2002 Practice Survey, the average family physician has 91.9 patient visits per week [6]. Given this high volume, even relatively small coding improvements can have dramatic effects on overall productivity. For example, a $5.00 increase in net revenue per visit over 45 weeks per year would result in over $20,000 per year in increased earnings.

Physician Practice Style

Every group practice is composed of physicians with different styles—the "tortoises" and the "hares" [7]. Additionally, complex, needy patients will gravitate toward physicians who spend more time on each visit, which further attenuates these style differences. It's no secret that certain types of patients gravitate toward certain physician styles, and physicians who have a higher percentage of complex patients should not be "punished" for this financially. The reality, however, is that seeing four level 3 visits per hour yields 2.68 RVUs, whereas seeing two level 4 visits per hour yields only 2.2 RVUs.

Part-Time or Full-time Employment Status

A full-time physician is likely to generate more annual RVUs than a part-time physician, and productivity targets need to be adjusted based on number of hours worked. It should also be taken into consideration that on an hour-by-hour basis, a part-time physician actually may be more productive than is a full-time physician [8]. Why is this? Contributing factors include the fact that it takes less energy to maintain a high productivity level for 20 hours per week than for 40 hours per week. Also, part-time physicians may have patient access issues that lead to a higher demand for their services when they are in clinic.

Scope of Practice

Family physicians provide a wide range of patient services that often include performing procedures and providing obstetric care. As previously noted, these services are reimbursed at variable RVU levels. A physician who practices obstetrics is likely to generate more annual RVUs than one who does not [3]. Similarly, outpatient surgical procedures tend to be reimbursed at a higher level than is cognitive care. In a group practice in which income is highly dependent on productivity, this can lead to physician desire to "game the system" by preferentially providing services that generate high RVUs and avoiding services that do not.

Patient Case Mix and Complexity of Care

Many physicians argue with some validity that productivity-based reimbursement does not equitably reimburse physicians who deal with patients with complex medical problems who require more time per visit.

This certainly is true if productivity is measured on a visit per hour basis. The RVU system does, at least partially, account for complexity of care and counseling time; thus, physicians need to have a thorough understanding of how to code visits based on time spent in counseling or in coordination of care. Accurate coding is essential, and physicians need training and feedback on coding accuracy to overcome this potential financial disadvantage.

Office Efficiency

How efficiently the practice operates can be a major determinant of physician productivity. Do physicians have adequate support staff to help them maximize their efficiency during patient care? A physician is the most expensive resource in a practice, and their time must be used wisely. Time spent going in and out of examination rooms for laboratory results, forms, and procedure supplies is simply wasted time. Investments in adequate staffing and examination room computers may be well worth the money spent if the physician can use his or her time more efficiently and see more patients.

Modifying Physician Productivity

"Well, says I, what's the use you learning to do right when it's troublesome to do right and ain't no trouble to do wrong, and the wages is just the same"?
—Huckleberry Finn [9]

So, just how do you herd a cat? Much has been said on various methods of motivating physicians to change their behavior; however no method has been found to be uniformly effective [10]. Greco and Eisenberg [11] describe six general methods for changing physician behavior: education, feedback, physician participation, administrative interventions, financial incentives, and financial penalties. Although these methods generally are described with respect to modifying quality of care or practice patterns, they also can be applied to other measures such as productivity. The one important caveat here that actually may make these methods more effective when applied to productivity is that in this case, there is personal risk (the individual physician's income is at stake). These methods are described briefly below with respect to how they can help influence physician productivity.

Education

Coding and billing education should be an integral part of any effort to increase physician productivity. Often physicians can dramatically increase their RVU revenue just by coding accurately for work they are already doing, even without any documentation changes. Regarding educational strategies, large group sessions are less effective than are individual and small group workshop sessions [10], and although these types of educational sessions are more labor and time intensive, they are likely to be worth the extra effort. A study by Kern et al [12] found that performance-based education measures were more effective than were didactic methods in altering physician practice patterns.

Feedback

Accurate and timely feedback is essential when trying to modify physician behavior. Comparison with peers is helpful. Sharing of individual productivity data among physicians may favorably increase productivity but decrease morale and collegiality. Another way to handle peer comparison but protect individual data is to show the physician his or her own productivity compared with clinic average, high, and low productivity values. Physician performance can be improved if privacy is protected, data are credible, and peers are used to provide feedback in a nonjudgmental way [13].

Physician Participation

Physicians should be involved in the design and implementation of any program that targets productivity improvement. The buy-in and use of "opinion leaders" (physicians having influence within the group) is essential, and these opinion leaders can help to motivate the group to succeed.

Administrative Interventions

This strategy refers to either creating barriers to undesired practices or reducing barriers to desired practices. As a physician leader, your goal should not be to increase the administrative hassles faced by your colleagues. Rather, you should seek to facilitate productivity increases by reducing barriers such as staffing shortages and redundant paperwork that dilute a physician's effectiveness during patient care.

Financial Incentives/Penalties

Efforts to increase productivity are more likely to be successful if there is a direct, tangible effect on physician income that is measurable and modifiable. It now is generally agreed that payment incentives do affect physician behavior [9]. An analysis by Gaynor and Pauley [14] found that as individual physician compensation changed from 0% to 100% dependent on productivity, physician productivity increased by 28%. However, the amount of incentive pay that will motivate a physician to change his or her behavior is variable from person to person, and physicians have an increasing tendency to value lifestyle over income. If the variable portion of a physician's income is not set at a level that will motivate him or her to change his or her behavior, it is unlikely that efforts to increase productivity will succeed.

Factors Influencing Success

Any efforts to increase productivity will be met with legitimate resistance if physicians do not feel that they have adequate support staff to increase the number of patients seen. It is important to note that this perceived staffing shortage may or may not actually be a factor in how difficult it is to increase productivity. Physicians often will cite lack of support as the reason that they are lower on the productivity scale or always running 30 minutes behind, when in actuality it may be their own personal interaction style with their patients that is the limiting factor. Observation and time studies can help to determine how to best intervene to help physicians meet their productivity goals.

Before motivating physicians to see more patients and making necessary scheduling changes to accomplish this (ie, changing the scheduling template to reduce visit length or increase session length) you need to assess whether you have patient capacity to accomplish the defined productivity goals. If not, either the goals will not be met or they will be met through a process know as "churning" (seeing the same patients over and over for unnecessary visits). This is not to say that productivity goals should not be set if patient volume is lacking. If productivity goals cannot be met by the current component of physicians, this is an argument for either increasing patient volume or decreasing physician FTEs, rather than abandoning productivity targets.

PHYSICIAN REIMBURSEMENT MODELS

Family Physician Salaries

Most physicians are interested in how their salary compares with that of their peers. According to an AAFP survey of 978 family physicians, the average (mean) family physician salary in 2001 was $135,800 and the median salary was $125,000 [15]. Salary data published by MGMA for both private and academic family physicians, with and without obstetrics, is listed in Table 3 [16].

Types of Reimbursement Models

The percentage of physicians who are self-employed in solo practice has been gradually declining. In 1984, 43% of physicians were employed in solo practice; however, by 1999 this number had decreased to 25% [5]. A 2003 survey of AAFP members revealed that only 18% of these physicians were employed in solo practice, whereas 64% were employed by a single-specialty or multispecialty group practice [17]. The following discussion applies to the increasing majority of physicians who are salaried employees and generally are members of a group practice or formal organization of some type.

TABLE 3.		
Family Physician Annual Compensation		
	Mean	**Median**
Private practice (2001 data)		
Family practice with obstetrics	$164,433	$150,290
Family practice without obstetrics	$159,679	$146,601
Academic practice (2002 data)		
Family practice with obstetrics	$154,393	$145,613
Family practice without obstetrics	$147,030	$144,409

It has been said that, "There are many mechanisms for paying physicians; some are good and some are bad. The three worst are fee-for-service, capitation, and salary" [9]. There are inherent problems with any of the existing physician compensation formulas and there is no perfect model. In general, physician salaries are based on one of three models: fixed salary, fixed salary plus variable incentive, or pure incentive. These models are explained further below.

Fixed Salary

Under this model, physician reimbursement is held at a fixed annual rate that does not have any variable component based on productivity or other measures. This model is becoming more rare because it does not provide any financial motivation for a physician to see more patients or implement any quality improvements.

Fixed Salary Plus Variable Incentive

This is becoming a common form of reimbursement model. A physician is guaranteed a fixed salary plus some type of variable component based on achieving performance objectives. "Negative incentives" refer to money that is withheld if goals are not met; "positive incentives" refer to money that is given if performance exceeds expected goals [18]. Careful attention must be paid to choosing the percentage of salary that is variable. If too little is variable, there will be insufficient motivation to increase productivity; if too much is variable, income may fluctuate at a level that is unacceptable to physicians.

Pure Incentive

This model can be not so fondly referred to as "eating what you kill" because it usually is totally dependent on productivity. It actually is similar to the situation faced by solo practitioners who own their practice. The inherent income variability of this model is likely to be less desirable to physicians who have chosen salaried employment over self-employment. In a group practice in which reimbursement is based on productivity alone, it can lead to intense competition for patient visits and also cause physicians' salaries to be unacceptably variable and dependent on factors over which they feel they have little control. It generally is extremely effective for increasing physician productivity, but at the expense of peer competition and potential overcoding for services.

INCENTIVE SYSTEM DESIGN

Deciding What to Measure and Reward

When designing an incentive system for employed physicians, it is important to consider what types of activities you want to reward. The system must be equitable, understandable, and compatible with the goals and mission of the organization. The most common incentive measure used is physician productivity. However, as previously mentioned, in a clinical setting in which a large percentage of patients are capitated, rewarding productivity may not make much sense financially. Regardless of payer mix, there may be many reasons for rewarding physicians for nonproductivity measures. Some of the more common components that may be included in an incentive system include (1) productivity, (2) patient panel size, (3) patient satisfaction, (4) quality measures (eg, HEDIS), (5) citizenship, (6) administration activities, and (7) resource use. It is essential that each component be measurable, modifiable, and reportable.

As one practice found, one factor to take into consideration is that basing compensation on too many components may have the effect of diluting the ability to change behavior in any one area [19]. For example, if multiple areas (productivity, patient satisfaction, HEDIS compliance, and so forth) are measured and financially compensated, the financial rewards for performing well in one area may be too small to incite the desired behavior change. Keeping the reimbursement formula simple and easily understandable also is critical.

Most group practices have sources of revenue from third-party payers that include capitated managed care contracts, discounted fee-for-service contracts, and RVU-based reimbursement. These contracts may or may not have their own quality measures built in as part of the practice's reimbursement. When deciding what types of incentives the group will use to reward individual physicians, these third-party payer measures need to be taken into consideration. Ultimately though, the group needs to decide on a method that is consistent with their own goals and values.

Determining Variable Percentage of Salary

The variable (at-risk) portion of salary can be any percentage of total salary, but in general should be high enough to motivate behavioral change yet low enough to avoid undue anxiety about income fluctuation. The majority of physician compensation methods have a guaranteed fixed component that ranges from 50% to 99% of total salary [20].

Productivity-Based Incentive System Design

If you choose to base all or part of your incentive system on productivity, you then need to decide how you are going to pay for this productivity. Options include paying the same amount for each RVU regardless of productivity level, paying incentive only when a certain target level is reached, or paying on a graduated scale based on productivity level. These models are explained below.

Straight Productivity Based

This model is the simplest to implement. It pays a fixed amount for each RVU generated, starting with the first RVU a physician earns and paying every subsequent RVU at the same rate.

Example: Physicians are paid $20 for each RVU earned. For a physician generating 4000 annual RVUs, this would lead to $80,000 in productivity-based income.

"Threshold" Model

This model does not begin incentive payments until a certain "threshold" productivity level is reached. This threshold may be based on fixed salary or a percentage of fixed salary. It protects the employer from losses incurred by low-productivity physicians. It is important that the threshold for receiving incentive payments be set at a level that physicians feel is achievable with reasonable productivity increases.

Example: Once a physician has reached a cumulative RVU total that is equal to 100% of the annual MGMA RVU benchmark, they are paid $30 for each subsequent RVU earned. With this model, the base salary needs to be set relatively high, and productivity-based incentive will be a relatively small percentage of the total salary.

Graduated Payment Model

With this model, physician clinical activity is reimbursed at variable levels depending on productivity. For example, if a physician generates 2.0 RVUs per hour, these RVUs will be reimbursed at a level that is different than that of a physician who generates 3.0 RVUs per hour. This model helps to account for the fact that lower-productivity physicians cost the group more money (in terms of lost revenue), but—unlike the threshold model—still allows for some reimbursement at all productivity levels.

Example: Physicians are paid $15 per RVU for the first 3000 annual RVUs earned, $20 per RVU for the next 1000 RVUs earned, and $25 per RVU for any subsequent RVUs earned.

Why would you want to consider using one of the more complex models? The advantage of using a threshold or graduated model is that they are more likely to motivate physicians to increase their productivity by selectively rewarding physicians who are more productive. The relative advantages and disadvantages of each incentive model are described in Table 4.

Setting an RVU Reimbursement Level

The selection of a compensation formula based on RVUs is greatly dependent on the individual group situation. Consideration needs to be given to the sources of revenue coming into the group, and also to the other expenses incurred by the group that need to be subsidized by clinical revenue. Obviously, the total amount being reimbursed as part of an incentive plan cannot be more than the amount of revenue coming in, or the amount of anticipated revenue after productivity increases.

Special Challenges Faced By Academic Departments

The determination of a total compensation package for physicians in an academic setting is an onerous, Herculean and sometimes mystical task. [21]

Anyone who has been involved in the design of a faculty salary plan can attest to the truth of this statement. Academic faculty have a wide variety of responsibilities including resident and medical student education, program administration, and research, all of which play a part in the many different hats a given faculty member may wear. Patient care is done in the time that is left over, and it is not unusual for faculty members to have varying amounts of clinical time, depending on their other responsibilities.

Developing an incentive program that rewards clinical productivity but does not compromise willingness to participate in academic activities

TABLE 4.
Comparison of Incentive Models

	Ease of Implementing	Protection from Losses Due to Lower Producers	Protection from Losses Due to Higher Producers	Ease of Comprehension by Physicians	Motivator for Increasing Productivity
Straight productivity	+++	+	++	+++	+
Threshold model	++	+++	+	++	++
Graduated model	+	+++	+	+	+++

can be a difficult task. One way to deal with this is to develop an incentive system that rewards physicians for clinical productivity and academic accomplishments. For example, "educational RVUs" can be given for medical student teaching, resident precepting, and other academic activities. "Research RVUs" can be used to encourage and reward research efforts such as grant awards and papers published. When determining the relative reimbursement for these activities, you must strike a delicate balance between generating enough clinical revenue to keep the department solvent and setting academic reimbursement high enough so that faculty will be encouraged to teach and publish without excessive concern about losing clinical incentive revenue. Funding for nonclinical RVUs may come from the academic institution, graduate medical education funds, and so forth, and also may need to be subsidized by clinical revenue.

Setting clinical productivity benchmarks for academic settings can be difficult. MGMA now is publishing salary and productivity benchmarks for academic practices, although sample sizes currently are too small to be of significant value. Setting benchmarks based on internal productivity is one solution—for example using the 75th percentile of annual department productivity, adjusted for clinical FTE status. Any productivity goals need to take into consideration the extra burden of medical student teaching, and for this reason holding academic practices to private physician productivity standards probably is not reasonable.

An example from the University of Michigan Department of Family Medicine illustrates one method of dealing with the complexity of an academic salary program. Faculty salaries are made up of the following components:

- Base salary—approximately 55% of total salary.
- Educational RVU incentive—approximately 10% of total salary. Academic activities such as medical student teaching, resident precepting, grand rounds presentations, and other lectures are reimbursed based on an internal RVU scale that assigns a numeric value to each of these activities based on time and complexity. Funding sources for this educational incentive program is subsidized by graduate medical education funding, medical school general funds, and clinical revenue.
- Clinical RVU incentive—approximately 35% of total salary. This currently is paid on a straight scale of $19 per RVU with no threshold. Plans are under way to move to a graduated reimbursement model that protects the department from losses due to low productivity while rewarding highly productive faculty at a relatively higher RVU rate.

Incentive Summary: Putting It All Together

In summary, when designing an incentive program, the following decisions need to be made:

What measures are to be included in the incentive program?
What percentage of salary is going to be "at risk" under the incentive program?
If reimbursing based on productivity, which method will be used?

Sample compensation plan #1:

Base salary—60%
Incentive (variable) component—40%
Productivity—20% (straight productivity based at $10 per RVU)
Patient panel size—10% (based on percentage of total clinic enrollees)
HEDIS compliance score—10% (determined by internal practice audit)

Sample compensation plan #2:

Base salary—50%
Incentive (variable) component —0%
Productivity—100% of incentive, using threshold model. Incentive payments begin once 50% of MGMA mean of 3980 (or 1990 RVUs) is reached. Compensation after 1990 is set at $30 per RVU.

Implementing an Incentive Plan–Essential Components

Anticipation

It is a fairly simple matter to calculate the financial impact of a new incentive system based on current productivity levels. However, it also is crucial to model various scenarios in which productivity increases and assess the financial impact on the practice/organization and also on individual physicians. The use of a spreadsheet program such as Microsoft Excel makes this a relatively easy task and ensures that the desired financial results will be maintained at various productivity levels.

Communication

Physicians need regular communication regarding any changes in salary structure, and ideally should be part of the decision-making process. Any potential barriers to increasing productivity such as staffing issues, lack of patient availability, and so forth need to be well thought out beforehand. These issues will be brought up and clearly formulated answers will be expected.

Data Integrity

The first thing that may happen upon implementing a new incentive system is that physicians will question the accuracy of the data being reported. Small mistakes will be interpreted as big problems. If there is truly a problem with data collection and reporting, do not proceed with an incentive model based on the data obtained until it is cleaned up.

Regular Feedback

Frequent and accurate feedback on individual clinical activity is critical to the success of any incentive program that includes plans to increase physician productivity. Feedback should be provided at least quarterly, possibly even monthly. Comparison with peers and with the individual's previous performance is helpful and should be included if possible.

Monitor Results and Celebrate Success

The implementation of a new incentive system is likely to be a source of anxiety and uncertainty for physicians. It is important to monitor the success of the system over its first year of operation and make certain that physicians are being rewarded equitably and as intended. Unintended consequences such as inequitable distribution or "gaming the system" need to be identified and corrected. If the intent of the system was to increase productivity, has this goal been accomplished? If so, celebrate this success. If not, this means that the bar was not set high enough to modify behavior and the payment rate or percentage of salary that is incentive based may need to be adjusted.

SUMMARY

> In physician payment, as in most other aspects of life, matters are never as good as we might hope but never as bad as we might fear. [9]

The medical profession has undergone significant changes in the last decade, including the method by which physicians are reimbursed for their work. Solo practice is being replaced by salaried employment, and many physicians are no longer "calling the shots" about how much they will be reimbursed or what this reimbursement will be based on. A thorough understanding of your organization's salary model and how productivity factors into the reimbursement equation is critical. The intent of this article is to provide an introduction to physician productivity and reimbursement, including factors for consideration when designing or evaluating an incentive system.

Many physicians mourn the perceived loss of control of being a salaried employee and feel that they have traded autonomy for security. The idealized Marcus Welby model that many of us grew up with is becoming increasingly rare. However, the idealism behind this model is still alive and well. Whether a physician has been in practice for several months or several decades, when all is said and done and it's just the physician and the patient behind a closed door, no financial arrangement has the power to truly alter that special relationship.

Key Points

- Physician productivity often is measured in terms of RVUs, which can be compared with internal or external benchmarks.
- When attempting to increase the productivity of an individual or group, careful attention must be paid to factors influencing physician productivity and behavior change.
- Employed family physicians commonly are reimbursed by a method that includes a base salary plus a variable component based on performance measures. These may include productivity, patient satisfaction, quality measures such as HEDIS, managed care panel size, citizenship, administrative activities, and resource use.
- Several incentive models can be used for reimbursing productivity based on RVUs earned. Examples are straight reimbursement, threshold, and graduated models.

References

[1] Jacob JA. Modest compensation gains for most doctors. American Medical News August 13, 2001:25.
[2] Johnson SE, Newton WP. Resource-based relative value units: a primer. Fam Med 2002;34(3):172–6.
[3] Medical Group Management Association. Physician compensation and production survey: 2002 report based on 2001 data. Englewood (CO): Medical Group Management Association; 2002.
[4] Goodson JD, Bierman AS, Fein O, et al. The future of capitation: the physician role in managing change in practice. J Gen Intern Med 2001;16(4):250–6.
[5] Centers for Medicare and Medicaid Services. The CMS chart series. Available at: www.cms.gov/charts. Accessed June 15, 2003.
[6] American Academy of Family Physicians. Table 13: average number of family physician visits per week and average number of patients in various settings, May 2003. Available at: www.aafp.org/x768.xml. Accessed July 1, 2003.
[7] Gillette RD. Turtles and rabbits: family physicians under time pressure. Family Practice Management 1999;6(4)April:21–4.
[8] Moore KJ. A productivity primer. Family Practice Management 2002;9(5)May:72–3.
[9] Robinson JC. Theory and practice in the design of physician payment incentives. The Milbank Quarterly 2001;79(2):149–77.
[10] Oxman AD, Thomson MA, Davis DA, et al. No magic bullets: a systematic review of 102 trials of interventions to improve professional practice. Can Med Assoc J 1995; 153(10):1423–31.
[11] Greco PJ, Eisenberg JM. Changing physicians' practices. N Engl J Med 1993; 329(17):1271–4.
[12] Kern DE, Harris WL, Boekeloo BO, et al. Use of an outpatient medical record audit to achieve educational objectives: changes in residents' performances over six years. J Gen Intern Med 1990;5(3):218–24.
[13] Nathanson P. Influencing physician practice patterns. Topics in Health Care Financing 1994;20(4):16–25.
[14] Gaynor M, Pauley MV. Compensation and production efficiency in partnerships: evidence from medical group practices. Journal of Political Economy 1990;98(3):544–73.
[15] American Academy of Family Physicians. Table 93: median and mean 2001 individual income before taxes (in thousands of dollars) of family physicians. Available at: www.aafp.org/x866.xml. Accessed June 15, 2003.

[16] Medical Group Management Association. Academic practice compensation and production survey for faculty and management: 2003 report based on 2002 data. Englewood (CO): Medical Group Management Association; 2002.

[17] American Academy of Family Physicians. Table 10: Practice arrangement of family physicians by chapter, January 1, 2003. Available at: www.aafp.org/x765.xml. Accessed June 20, 2003.

[18] Moore KJ. Evaluating bonuses and incentives: the basics. Family Practice Management 1999;6(6)June:53–5.

[19] Colodny CS. Implementing a new plan to compensate physicians. Family Practice Management 2000;7(8)Sept.:29–40.

[20] Greenfield WR. In search of an effective physician compensation formula. Family Practice Management 1998;5(9)Oct.:50–7.

[21] Krohn A. Provider compensation in the academic medical practice: one revolution: managing the academic medical practice in an era of rapid change. Englewood (CO): Medical Group Management Association; 1997.

Address reprint requests to

Jean M. Malouin MD, MPH
Department of Family Medicine
University of Michigan
1500 E. Medical Center Drive
L2003 Women's Hospital
Ann Arbor MI 48109-0239

e-mail: jskratek@umich.edu

PROFESSIONAL AND PRACTICE MANAGEMENT SKILLS 1522–5720/03 $15.00 + .00

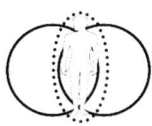

IMPROVING OFFICE OPERATIONS

Randall T. Forsch, MD, MPH

Family physicians now share a concern that they work much harder to maintain incomes or even to stay in practice. Although a recent study [1] suggests that the number of visits per week has declined, incomes remained constant or even increased due to efficiency measures or improvements. In 2002, the average family physician in the United States had 91.9 office visits, 9.7 hospital visits, 3.2 nursing home visits, and 0.3 house calls per week. In addition, the physician weekly supervised 5.0 home health care, 9.7 nursing home, and 1.4 hospice patients [2]. What if that did not generate the necessary weekly revenue to maintain a profitable practice and comfortable income or even keep the clinic doors open?

One solution might be to provide more patient care. How might this be done? Although other patient care settings are more dependent on specific health situations—that is, a severity of illness necessitating hospital admission—the outpatient clinic is the venue in which the physician has the most control of patient visits. A modest increase in patient volume with an attendant increase in billable services can be accomplished most easily by increasing the efficiency of the clinic. On the other hand, increasing patient volume in the clinic may lead to lower rates of preventive services delivery, lower patient satisfaction, and less positive doctor–patient relationships at the cost of efficiency [3]. Further, what worked to increase efficiency and productivity at a clinic in the past might not work today.

If your office is not faced with a financial crisis, should you still consider increasing efficiency? The resounding answer is "Yes!" Increased efficiency in the office makes everyone's job easier and more satisfying by increasing clinic revenue; quality of care; and satisfaction of patients, staff, and physicians. This article explores office efficiency, describes seven strategic themes for increasing efficiency, and demonstrates methods to measure and improve efficiency. Each section has something to offer, even though it may not fit your practice today or meet all three goals at once.

From the Department of Family Medicine, University of Michigan Medical Director, Chelsea Family Practice Center, Chelsea, Michigan

EFFICIENCY

In health care economics, the efficiency is "the return or output achieved for a given level of input or resource" [4]. In the clinical setting, efficiency can be considered a measure of how well tasks are accomplished with resources allotted to them.

The goal of efficiency in the clinic is to maximize clinical productivity while minimizing the waste of resources. A good way to think of this is to consider capacity and work in the context of the physician's time while providing care to patients during a clinic session. Capacity is the maximum amount of resources (time) that can be provided by a resource (physician). Thus, physician time can be used either productively for work (patient care) or wasted (nonpatient care), but the total time cannot be increased. When all of a physician's time is used for patient care, then maximal productivity is achieved and efficiency is considered high. The clinical resources (ie, space, money, personnel, and information) may vary, as may the tasks, but all must be used efficiently to meet the needs of the patient.

The definition of efficiency varies with audience. For the physician example above, the definition of efficiency is "maximizing the time spent providing patient care." This allows the most attention to be focused on patient health needs as well as for the most total patient care to be provided. Interestingly, the same holds true for the individual patient, who frequently thinks that the only time that matters during the entire visit to the clinic is that spent face-to-face with the physician [5]. However, if the time of the entire clinic visit is considered, other members of the health care team, such as clerks and nurses, and the time needed to perform their essential tasks should be considered with regard to efficiency.

As noted above, the determination of efficiency requires the measurement of the use of resources to produce a given result or accomplish a task. This measurement can be made; however, a determination of whether efficiency has been achieved still needs to be made. One way to do this would be to measure the clinic's result once, measure it again, and compare the two results. The difference between the two measurements can demonstrate change and, hopefully, improvement, and is a great place to start. It does not, however, provide the comparative data necessary to determine maximal efficiency and compete in the health care market.

One common method of measuring efficiency is to compare individual results with those of peers. These peer results, called benchmarks, serve as a standard by which a true comparison may be made [6]. These results may be whole numbers such as clinic visits per year or ratios such as visits per medical assistant. The title "best practice" goes to the site, usually with the most efficient clinical operation, that has the best results and sets a benchmark standard. The peers used for comparison may be within the same clinic, health system, or specialty. To be most useful, they should be peers faced with the same clinical challenges and performing the same tasks with the same or similar resources. To compare a private practice with an academic practice or a rural fee-for-service clinic with an urban managed-care practice would not be as useful. Currently, the most commonly used benchmarking data comes from national organizations, such as the Medical Group Management Association (MGMA) and the American Academy of Family Physicians (AAFP), who report members' results across specialty and practice settings.

CLINICAL RESOURCES FOR THE OFFICE VISIT

Before you can seek ways to be more efficient in clinical operations, you need to consider what clinical resources are required and how best to use them to efficiently provide care for your patients. Each of these resources has efficiency that can be measured and potentially improved.

It is useful to consider the patient visit in terms that Einstein would use—that is, as the flow of the patient through space and time. From 1999 MGMA data [7], the average full-time family physician had 1528 feet allocated in the clinic. In this space are the support staff; medical assistants; nurses; reception area; medical records shelves; light fixtures; bathrooms; storage areas; staff desks; hallways; emergency exits; physician offices; waiting rooms; and two or three dedicated examination and treatment rooms with their examination tables, desks, and equipment. Physician support staff must have space to do their tasks. As is apparent, the patient's use of space is limited to the hallways, waiting room, and examination/treatment room during the visit and the checkout area after the visit. Nonvisit-based care can be provided outside of the clinic (eg, over the telephone or by e-mail) and may be very beneficial to patients—especially managed care patients—but will greatly impact the other variable, time.

The AAFP reported that in 2002, the average clinic-based family physician worked 50.1 hours per week, with 40.9 hours spent in direct patient care. Further, the average number of weeks per year practiced was 47.2, leading to a total of 1930 direct patient care hours [8]. Clearly, much physician time is spent taking care of patients. Those hours can be multiplied by the number of physician support staff at a clinic and a large and expensive number results. The staff that use this time usually have direct patient contact such as the receptionist, medical assistant, and nurse, but also includes the clerks working in medical records, billing, and referrals and those staff doing housekeeping and physical plant maintenance.

Until the second half of the twentieth century, the typical family practice office had a staff of two: the physician and a nurse. All the tasks of patient care and running the office were divided between the two, including patient flow, billing, and housekeeping. Overhead could be kept low, due to the fact that doctors performed house calls. Since that time, more specialized staff with diverse skills have been required, mostly with regard to the business of medicine. It is typical for a family practice office to have about 3.5 full-time equivalent (FTE) staff to support a 1.0 FTE physician. This breaks down to 2.0 FTE front desk staff, 1.0 FTE medical assistants, and 0.5 FTE nurse. Think of the FTE positions as representative of the clusters of tasks necessary to run the clinic. In that way, it may make sense to have "parts" of positions to support a physician that actually can be a single full-time position.

SEVEN STRATEGIC THEMES FOR IMPROVING CLINICAL EFFICIENCY

Clinical efficiency may be increased in many ways. Ask experienced clinicians and they will share tricks that they use to "save time" or be more efficient. For example, it has been determined that wearing a stethoscope around the neck in the traditional manner rather than the "cool" draped-around-the neck manner as depicted on medical TV shows is more efficient [9]. Regardless of the setting, the seven major themes below (time management, communication, delegation of tasks, teamwork, simplification and standardization, information flow, and maximization of the visit) all have something to offer. As you read through them and the associated suggested best practices, think about your current practice and whether these suggestions might make your clinic more efficient.

Time Management

Time is money. This phrase has been used by bosses to motivate workers for years. It should motivate you as well. If you make the most of all your time in clinic, the yield will be great. By "doing today's work today"—a phrase encouraged by the Institute for Health Care Improvement—physicians can keep on top of tasks and hopefully not fall behind [10]. Remember that you, the physician are the rate-limiting step with regard to patient flow in the clinic. Your time is a limited resource; how do you want to use it?

1. Stay on time. Nearly half of Americans recently polled said that they typically wait 20 minutes or more in the waiting room, but only 15% said that was acceptable [11]. Starting your clinic session on time at the very least allows you to begin clinic on schedule. Did you know that a patient's opinion of the care provided by the physician varies inversely with length of wait in the office [12]? Watch the clock to remind yourself of how much time you have before the next visit. Have your medical assistant also keep track of your time and prompt you as appropriate. This sometimes can save you from the "oh, by the way" patient who does not want the visit to ever end.

2. Use your time. Although we all need to have fun at work, try to avoid wasting time getting a cup of coffee or with idle chatter. If you have time before the next patient, dictate the note while the information is fresh. Some physicians with the technology are even documenting the visit in the presence of the patient! Do not put off

work for later—do it now. You'll be happier at the end of the day when you can go home without a stack of charts waiting.

3. Use your schedule. A significant variation occurs in how clinical schedules are kept. (For more information on this topic, see Zazove's article elsewhere in this issue) The amount of time reserved for the patient visit must match that needed to provide the necessary care. Regardless of the scheduling system, there are ways for the physician to use it efficiently. For example, if you schedule health maintenance examination (HME) visits for 30 minutes, an urgent-care appointment can be scheduled at the same time and seen either while the HME patient is being checked in or while he or she is undressing and putting on a gown. Another way that physicians can manage their schedule is by appropriately lengthening the time between follow-up visits. For example, if a physician routinely sees stable chronic disease patients such as those with diabetes mellitus or hypertension every 3 months, a change to every 4 months would open up one additional visit for another patient per year. Multiply this extra visit by the number of chronic disease patients in the practice and the increased access is significant. This simple move would not significantly impact the care of the stable chronic disease patient, but would significantly increase access for others.

Communication

You communicate with many people every day; if you make sure that you do it effectively, your office efficiency will increase. Improve communication with your staff and they will meet the patients' and your needs better. Improve your communication skills with patients and you'll save time with decreased callbacks for explanations of instructions, medication changes, or care plans. Improve your communication with external entities such as pharmacies and insurance companies, and you'll have less paperwork to handle.

1. Write legibly. If someone cannot read your writing, mistakes can happen. The person unable to read your writing has to clarify it with you, which adds a task for both of you and takes time. If you cannot write legibly, print. If you cannot do that, find technology—such as check off forms, printed prescriptions, or the like—to make your message clear and understandable.

2. Let the patient talk. Patients' satisfaction increases when they believe their physician listens. Open the patient visit with a smile, a handshake, and "What can I do for you today"? This open-ended question can save time by letting patients tell you the reason for the visit, their concerns and their agenda from the onset. Frequently, most of the information you need comes forth spontaneously. Most physicians are reluctant to do this for fear it will open a pandora's

box of unlimited questions. However, if left to talk without interruption, most patients only speak for 3 to 4 minutes. You then can assess their information, ask more directed questions, and continue the visit as appropriate. A 1999 study showed that only 28% of initial concerns were completed because of redirection by the physician [13]. This led to missed opportunities to gather important data and also to feelings of dissatisfaction and unmet needs by the patient.

3. Follow Sir William Olser's advice: "Save the fleeting Minute, learn gracefully to dodge the bore" [14]. The risk of the open-ended approach is getting caught by the patient with the literal laundry list of concerns and questions. Keeping in mind that many patients need your expertise on a given day and that your expertise can help sort through the list to address clinically relevant issues, negotiate with the patient about what concerns will be addressed during the current visit. In one study, 2.7 clinical problems were addressed on average and each additional problem lengthened the visit by 2.5 minutes [15]. Other issues can be dealt with at another time, via correspondence or by staff.

4. Localization. At any given time, your staff needs to know where you are and you need to know where you need to be. Keep an up-to-date daily calendar and personal schedule that staff can reference. Use high technology such as pagers and wireless telephones to be kept available. Use colored flags or the like outside of clinic rooms to identify rooms for your patients when you share a hall with another provider. A flag with a chart underneath lets you know where to go; if the chart is gone, your staff knows that you are with the patient. This low-tech system can be effective. By knowing where you should be and by being there, time spent searching is avoided.

Delegation of Tasks

One of the most important things that interns learn in the clinic is that the new MD that follows their name also stands for "Must Delegate." All too frequently they are still in the medical student mode of doing all clinical tasks for themselves, including setting up rooms and doing electrocardiograms. Although this method has educational usefulness, it is inefficient. Too much valuable time can be wasted by the physician doing tasks that should be handled by others. It is imperative that tasks requiring nonphysician skills are delegated to others. This does not mean that the tasks are "below" physicians and should never be performed by them. That would go against the concept of teamwork. It does mean, however, that limited resources, such as physician or nurse time, should not be diverted from their primary and most effective purpose.

1. Learn to delegate. The physician is the most expensive and valuable worker at the clinic. Physician expertise needs to be used for patient care. This applies to all staff and tasks; have the task at hand

performed by the least expensive staff member who can complete it successfully.

2. Share your patients. The typical family physician generates the majority of annual revenue in the clinic, not in the hospital. Because of this and the demands of call, inpatient care frequently is shared by physicians. The issue is time and how to use it efficiently. Is it worth the hour driving to the hospital to round on one or two patients, or would that time be more efficiently spent in the clinic? The latter is usually true. The more common practice is to have a member of the physician's call group round on the group's inpatients, thereby increasing the efficiency of the time spent rounding in the hospital for the one and adding those travel hours to patient care in the clinic to the group. The extreme position is to eliminate inpatient care altogether and use a hospitalist or a different group for inpatient coverage.

Teamwork

Teamwork is imperative for efficient clinical operations. Without teamwork, the office will run, but rarely succeed. This applies to all members of the team, from the person who greets the patient at the door, through the physician, to the person who checks the patient out. It is the responsibility of the physician to be a role model for teamwork and to act like the coach, not the owner. If a physician is willing to help staff with their tasks (eg, phoning in prescriptions when the nurse is educating a patient, rather than just sitting down and drinking a cup of coffee while waiting for the next patient), the return will be great. The following illustrate the benefits of teamwork on clinical efficiency.

1. Have a mission. Everyone in the office needs to share the same vision—that is, "Our vision is to inspire a healthy community, one patient at a time,"—and the same mission—that is, "We at the Chelsea Health Center are committed to working as a team to promote the well being of our patients, families, and staff by providing compassionate, quality care using the building blocks of research and education." Although a small office may have a straightforward mission agreed on by all, those of larger or more heterogeneous practices frequently require much more discussion and participation. Vision and mission statements are best developed by the physicians and staff so that everyone feels invested and represented. Frequently, an outside facilitator is required to get the process under way, keep the group on task, and maintain balance.

2. Cross-training. Staff should be cross-trained on the clinical tasks that are expected to require extra help (eg, scheduling patients) and are relatively easy to learn. By having staff who are able to cross-cover and understand the importance of tasks, time will not be wasted waiting for the one and only person who is able to perform the task.

3. Huddle up. A 5-minute meeting or team huddle before the clinic session accomplishes many things. It lets team members look at the day's work together and anticipate needs, head off problems, and organize resources to meet the day. Support staff then will know, before the day's visits, which setup is needed for a procedure, to pull an emergency room report, or to run the office laboratory immediately when the patient presents, all saving time. Most importantly, a group meeting promotes the sense of team that makes teamwork easier to accomplish.

Simplification and Standardization

The military is credited with the K.I.S.S. system useful for operational issues. K.I.S.S. stands for "Keep It Simple, Stupid" an effective phrase to keep in mind for many settings, including the clinical office. The concept is that because people like simple things, the complexity of a task or system should be limited. Standardization is another way to simplify a task or system. Being able to do most tasks in most places the same way increases efficiency. An advantage to both simplification and standardization is that both promote a clinical system offering fewer opportunities for mistakes and waste.

1. Standardize schedules. By keeping the clinic schedule for all providers standardized, mistakes are more difficult to make. For example, if the staff know that HME visits take 30 minutes, it is much more difficult to try to schedule one inappropriately to the frustration of both physician and patient.
2. Standardize rooms. Make each examination room identical and interchangeable. Specialization of rooms for specific purposes only leads to bottlenecks when demand exceeds capacity. Every room should be equipped to handle most of the patient visits. Specialized materials and equipment should be mobile so that they can be taken into the room when needed.
3. Make tasks simple. Nobody likes to make a mistake or fail to accomplish a task. Make sure that your clinic systems are in place to make it easy to perform the task at hand successfully. This can be accomplished through education about the task, practice of the task, or by continuously reviewing the system around the task to ensure that the best and most simple method is being used. For example, each examination room should have all the forms needed for the visit (eg, laboratory requisition or referral forms), rather than keeping the forms centralized. By having the forms in the room, the step of obtaining the needed form by physically leaving the room or asking someone to obtain it is eliminated. This simplification also saves time for both the physician and the support staff and may well head off the mistakes that lead to adverse events [16].

4. Simplify documentation. Much of patient care follows a standard pattern. Use simple, standardized forms to document important information. A history is obtained from the patient to characterize the presenting complaint, the patient is examined to further delineate and diagnosis the complaint, and finally a workup and treatment plan are recommended. For many visits, the physician follows a standard pattern for the history, physical, and treatment plan. Dictation templates simplify the documentation process. A great place to start this process is with the routine HME, the content of which varies mostly on age of the patient. Physicians can use a worksheet (Fig. 1) that allows them to record the important findings and also prompts them with regard to important HME components, screening tests, and patient education topics. Also, consider dictating telephone calls so that loose notes do not need to be found and attached to the chart.

Information Flow

Physicians deal with ever-increasing clinical information daily, which at times can be overwhelming. This information needs to be managed to efficiently provide the high quality of care that physicians and their patients desire and deserve.

1. Be ready. Have visit-related information such as visit notes, laboratory studies, and roentgenograms ready before the visit. This allows the physician to prepare and eliminates wasted time waiting for results. Have the materials needed for the visit (eg, laboratory order sheet or referral sheet) with the chart at the start of the visit so that they can be completed readily. Also, have ready access, either online or preprinted, to patient education materials. All this preparation will save time that can be devoted to patient care.
2. Use information technology (IT). Medicine continues to be more complex. Much of the complexity involves clinically relevant information. Consider having either hardwired or wireless computer access in each examination room, which will save paper and offer instant access to legible clinical notes and studies and to searchable clinical information references, calculators, web pages, and e-mail. (For more information on IT in clinical practice, please see Ebell's article elsewhere in this issue.)
3. Keep track of information. It is imperative that clinical information is monitored so that appropriate decision making and follow-up occurs. Every physician has heard the story of the ignored or missed result that led to an unfortunate result for the patient and a malpractice suit for the physician. All physicians have their own clinical information tracking method, usually by lists generated at the time of the visit. Frequently, the tracking task is delegated to a nurse who notifies the physician of abnormal results so that an

FIGURE 1.
HME template.

Chelsea Family Practice HME Template

Name:

Reg. #:

CC: (optional)

HPI: (optional)
Location, Quality, Severity, Duration, Timing, Context
Modifiers, Assoc. signs/symptoms

Routine HME. No concerns and chronic conditions stable except as noted below.

ROS: (need 10)
Negative x 10 systems except as noted below.

NI	Abn		NI	Abn	
☐	☐	Constitutional	☐	☐	Musc/Skel
☐	☐	Eyes	☐	☐	Skin
☐	☐	ENT	☐	☐	Neuro
☐	☐	Resp	☐	☐	Psych
☐	☐	CV	☐	☐	Endo
☐	☐	GI	☐	☐	Heme/Lymph
☐	☐	GU	☐	☐	All/Immun

PMFSHx: (need all three)
Updated. See face sheet and genogram.

Describe:

PHYSICAL EXAM: (2 bullets from 9 systems)

NI	Abn	Constitutional	BP	Weight	P	R	T	HT
		Need 3 vitals->						
☐	☐	Appearance						

NI	Abn	EYES
☐	☐	Conjunctivitis & lids
☐	☐	Pupils
		ENT
☐	☐	External ears & nose
☐	☐	Mouth
☐	☐	Mucous Membrane
☐	☐	Pharynx
		NECK
☐	☐	Neck
☐	☐	Thyroid
		RESPIRATORY
☐	☐	Auscultation
☐	☐	Effort
		CARDIOVASCULAR
☐	☐	Auscultation
☐	☐	Pedal pulses
☐	☐	Extremities (edema)
		GI
☐	☐	Abdomen
☐	☐	Liver & spleen
		LYMPHATIC
☐	☐	Neck
☐	☐	Groin

NI	Abn	MUSCULOSKELETAL
☐	☐	Gait & posture
☐	☐	Clubbing or cyanosis
		SKIN
☐	☐	Inspection
☐	☐	Palpation
		PSYCHIATRIC
☐	☐	Orientation
☐	☐	Mood & Effect

Must dictate if done:

NI	Abn	BREAST
☐	☐	Inspection
☐	☐	Breast & axilla palpation
		PELVIC (female)
☐	☐	Ext. genitalia & vagina
☐	☐	Uterus
☐	☐	Adnexa
☐	☐	Cervix
☐	☐	Urethra & Meatus
☐	☐	Bladder
☐	☐	Anus/Perineum
		GU
☐	☐	Anus
☐	☐	Penis/Scrotum
☐	☐	Prostate

Labs Reviewed / X-rays Reviewed / I personally visualized image, EKG, or specimen

ASSESSMENT: Must dictate
1) Health Maintenance
2) Pap
   Imms (Td, Flu, Pneumovax, HepB)
   Labs (CHD, PSA, LFT's, HbA1C, creat, Microalb/creat)
3) Colonoscopy or Flex Sig >50yo (>40 or risk factors)
   Mammo >50yo (discuss >40 if risk factors)
   Osteoporosis prevention (DEXA, Calcium)
4) Diet, exercise, and healthy behaviors discussed

appropriate plan is developed. The success of these systems varies on the diligence and timeliness of those involved, so both the people and the system need to be reliable.

4. Ticklers. We all want to provide quality care to our patients. Sometimes the most important care gets buried under the mundane. This happens when the chief complaint of a visit is so significant that all our attention and energy needs to be focused on it alone. It also happens when the patient is an "infrequent flier" and underuses your services. Regardless of cause, important screening tests frequently are not ordered in a timely manner. To avoid this, a tickler system needs to be in place that will prompt the physician, patient, or both about the test. Commonly, lists for telephone calls or postcards are used. At the University of Michigan Department of Family Medicine, a trial is underway of "Clinfotracker," a software system that can, among other things, prompt and remind the physician about screening tests appropriate for age and diagnosis [17]. For example, when a 60-year-old female diabetic presents for a visit, Clinfotracker will prompt the physician about hemoglobin A_{1c}, retinal screening, diabetic foot examination, and microalbuminuria screening, as well as mammography and colonoscopy. Regardless of the method of tracking, clinical efficiency will increase when ticklers are used.

Maximization of the Visit

Most physicians are being driven to be more productive regardless of their setting. One way to accomplish this is to do more for a patient at the visit. If performed efficiently, everyone wins. Patient satisfaction and physician productivity increase when today's visit is maximized. Further, access for other patients increases when multiple clinical issues are addressed or dealt with during a single visit. A great example of maximizing the visit is freezing an actinic keratosis that was identified during an HME visit. The procedure takes little time and doing it immediately takes care of the problem, adds productivity to the time allotted to the visit, and saves a visit for another patient in the future. Use your time wisely and be careful that you do not do too much for the current patient and cause unnecessary waits for other patients.

1. Do today's work today. The Institute for Health care Improvement emphasizes this point and the efficiency it offers. By not putting off tasks, you start each day with a clean slate rather than a workload that looks difficult to begin with and becomes unmanageable with time. With regard to patient care, make that referral, dictate that letter, order that test, and do that procedure today.
2. Keep an agenda. Although the patient has his or her agenda that you can solicit, keep your own with regard to the visit. By making sure

that the patient is up to date with important health maintenance issues such as immunizations and screening tests and addressing these issues at the visit, you again are improving patient care.

3. Group visits. Family physicians already add value to patient visits by taking care of a secondary patient almost 20% percent of the time [18]. The next step, group visits, increase efficiency by distributing more of the physician effort to more patients per unit of time. Group visits maximize physician time by taking care of multiple patients concurrently during a given time period. Drop-in group medical appointments are designated 90-minute appointments co-led by a physician and behavioral health professional. Cooperative health care clinics are 2-hour scheduled appointments run by a physician and nurse for a specific disease, such as diabetes mellitus or metabolic syndrome. A good discussion of group visits may be found in Houck et al [19].

A TOOL FOR IMPROVING EFFICIENCY IN THE CLINIC

Efficiency in the clinic frequently can be improved by a simple process that will yield obvious results. Adoption of a new technology— for example, dictating notes instead of handwriting them—is a good example. Frequently, however, the process is not that simple or the results are not that obvious to assess. Special skills and tools are required to make the change to improve efficiency in the clinic and measure its results. This section describes common techniques that can be used in any clinic to improve almost any problem.

In the clinic, efficiency and quality go hand in hand with regard to patient care and clinical operations, and much work has been done since the 1990s to develop processes for improvement. Quality improvement (QI) is a method of continuously assessing processes and making them more effective. W. Edwards Deming, PhD, revolutionized management theories in the United States and Japan with the following principles: (1) focus on customers' needs and desires; (2) continuously improve all processes; (3) involve the entire organization, not just management, in seeking quality; and (4) use data and a diverse team to address the problem and develop the solution [20]. These principles have been used successfully in improving processes for organizations great and small. In the medical office, they can be applied to improve patient flow, decrease wait time, and increase patient satisfaction, as well as many other processes.

With QI, you first must identify your goal (usually improving a process or solving a problem), the measurable criteria with which you will determine improvement, and the changes you plan to make to accomplish the improvement. In its simplest form, the QI process follows the four-part "plan–do–study–act" cycle. During the "Plan" phase, a team analyzes the process, makes determinations as to potential effective changes, and plans for making the improvement. "Do" puts a small-scale trial into motion. "Study" checks to see if the trial is working. Finally, "Act" involves implementing a successful change on a larger scale or continuing work on finding one.

Many physicians wonder where to begin with QI because they can find many problems within their clinics that should be addressed for improvement. Here are some recommendations to the best sources who can help you pinpoint those issues needing QI attention. First, ask your customers what can be improved with formal surveys or informal questions. Your customers are not only your patients, but also your staff and colleagues who will know what needs improvement. Another method is to look for "waste" in the clinic from a variety of points of view. For example, is bottlenecking occurring because of the current process that wastes patient and staff time? Internal reviews using patient complaint cards or chart audits can identify issues that need improvement, such as immunization rates and other Health Employer Data Information Set criteria. All physicians are part of larger organizations that monitor their practice; the third-party payers frequently send information comparing your profile to other similar family physicians. If you are an outlier, it might point to a place to focus QI efforts. Explore "best practices" or what other clinics have done well and see if it makes sense for you to adopt their processes. Once you have a list of potential problems or issues to address, prioritize them based on how fixable and measurable they are and how much addressing them will improve the processes in your clinic.

Once you identify the problem to be addressed, it is time to assemble a QI team. This team needs support and resources dedicated to them from clinic leadership. The task at hand needs to be "chartered"; that is, establishing what is to be done and why it is important. By establishing the QI team's charter—which includes a description of the process to addressed, the reason for making improvement, how improvement will be demonstrated, who is impacted by changes, a timeline, available resources for task, and a communication plan with leadership—a clear plan is communicated. Team members are best chosen from those who have a stake in the process to be improved and should be volunteers with diverse job functions. Keep the group small—six to eight members—and identify a team leader to focus on the mechanics of the task (schedule, content of meetings, and record keeping) and a facilitator whose task is to focus on the process (how team members participate and interact). Every team member is treated as an equal and must participate. Education should be available about the QI process, especially the common FOCUS-PDSA model (Box 1)[21]. (For an excellent discussion of a team approach to QI, see Schwarz et al [21].)

Once the team is clear on the task at hand and has the resources (including knowledge, time, and support) necessary to succeed, the FOCUS-PDSA model can be implemented. "Focus" and "Organize" have been accomplished already; the next step is to "Clarify" the current process and gather baseline data. Good data are essential to the QI process and what is to be collected needs to be specific. Data should include benchmarks as well as that from your own clinic. "Understand" the sources of process variation by flowcharting the entire process from

> ## Box 1. FOCUS-PDSA Model [21]
>
> Find a clinical process to improve
> Organize the diverse team and its resources
> Clarify knowledge about the current process (analyze baseline data)
> Understand sources of variation and clarify steps in the process
> Select an improvement or intervention
> Plan how you will implement the intervention
> Do it (carry out the change, preferably on a small scale)
> Study the process to see whether the intervention created improvement
> Act on what you have learned, which may mean either implementing the change on a larger scale, starting over, or tackling a new area of improvement

beginning to end, identifying the major steps in the proper sequence to show the flow of the process. Fig. 2 shows a flowchart of a simple process involving a medical assistant and immunizations with nine steps [21]. Flowcharting can clarify the process and help to identify problem areas.

At this point, the QI team has a charter, baseline data, and a flowchart with identified steps that can be improved. They should "Select" a small-scale intervention to improve the process using the above resources. "Plan" is the stage at which the intervention is planned, which can be challenging if changing a significant process. "Do" is when the planned intervention is executed, whereas "Study" evaluates its results to compare with baseline data. "Act" is the stage at which everything is pulled together and a decision is made to adopt the small-scale intervention for the whole clinic or to do more study to find a better solution. The next challenges are to hold the gains and to continue the QI process, which are beyond the scope of this article [22]. Our experience at the University of Michigan Department of Family Medicine with successful and unsuccessful efforts in QI is well documented in the 1998 Zazove and Klinkman article [23]. The FOCUS-PDSA process-improvement model can be useful in improving clinical issues great and small. Give it a try!

MAKING OPERATIONS EFFICIENT

This article began with a discussion of the definition of efficiency in the clinic, described how to measure it, and reviewed the clinical resources available to accomplish clinical tasks. The seven strategic themes in which efficiency can be found were emphasized and examples of ways to achieve it were given. Finally, the QI technique for measuring and improving clinic operations was illustrated.

This information should be useful in most family medicine clinics and also should be doable. Sometimes, however, leaders at clinics do not believe they have the resources available, such as time and money, to look

FIGURE 2.
Flowchart of medical assistant (MA) role with pediatric immunization. A parallelogram is the starting point; a rectangle, a task; a diamond, a decision point; and an oval, the endpoint.

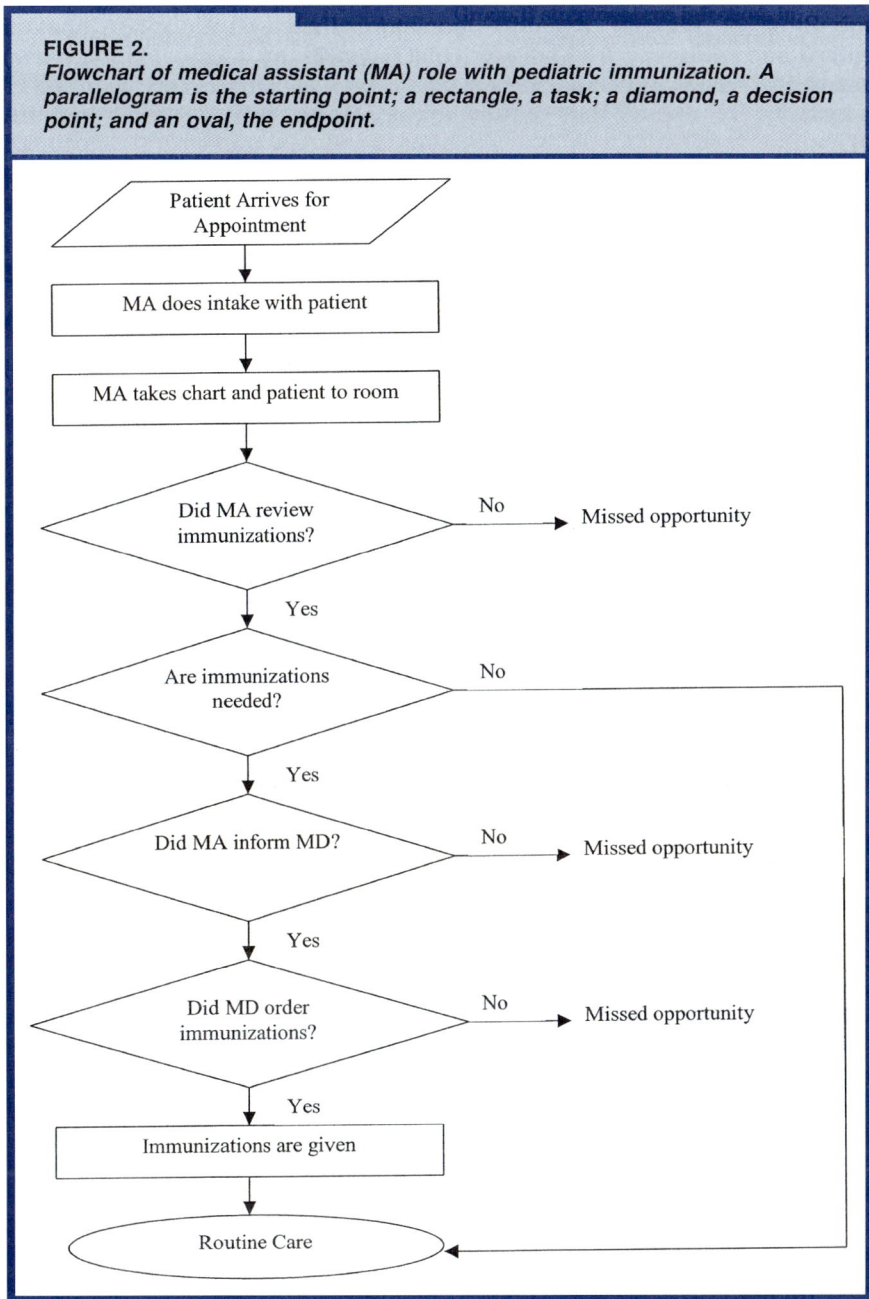

at a problem and work for an improvement. They then have to determine for themselves what the return on investment will be by allocating resources to address the clinical problem. If they truly cannot allocate dedicated resources, then the following suggestions may help. In the case of a lack of funds, look at how "best practices" have addressed the problem and adopt their methods if possible. In the case of a lack of time to dedicate to the problem, find a willing consultant to come in and help you with the problem. Although this may be expensive, the consultant should bring a broad knowledge base and perspective that can greatly aid the QI process.

Key Points

- Use benchmarks and best practices to measure your clinical efficiency.
- Do today's work today.
- Let the patient talk, within reason.
- Delegate to team members, but still be part of the team.
- Have a vision and mission statement to promote teamwork.
- Simplify and standardize to increase efficiency and decrease waste and mistakes.
- Make quality improvement part of your standard practice.

APPENDIX

Resources

American Academy of Family Practice (AAFP): www.aafp.org. This site provides data and information about family physicians and links to their Family Practice Management journal.

Institute for Health care Improvement (IHI): www.ihi.org. This site introduces the organization's concepts and provides resources for improving clinical operations. Be sure to look at their Idealized

Joint Commission on Accreditation for Health care Organizations: www.jcaho.org. This site provides information on standards and quality at the hospital and health system level, yet much is useful in the clinic.

Medical Group Management Association (MGMA): www.mgma.com. The most commonly used source for benchmarking data; requires membership for access.

References

[1] Weeks WB, Wallace AE. Time and money: a retrospective evaluation of the inputs, outputs, efficiency, and incomes of physicians. Arch Intern Med 2003;163(8):944–8.

[2] American Academy of Family Physicians. Average number of family physician visits per week and average number of patients in various settings, May 2002. Available at: www.aafp.org/x768.xml.

[3] Zyanski SJ, Stange KC, Langa D, et al. Trade-offs in high-volume primary care practice. J Fam Pract 1998;46(5):397–402.

[4] Griffith JR. The well-managed healthcare organization. 4th edition. Chicago: AUPHA Press; 1999. p. 674.

[5] Time spent with patients. Available at: www.docrates.net/QuickReport/timespent.htm.

[6] Witt MJ. Improving group practice performance with benchmarking. Health Financial Management 2001;55(2):67–70.

[7] Medical Group Management Association. Cost survey: 2000 report based on 1999 data. Englewood (CO): Medical Group Management Association; 2002. p. 131.

[8] Average number of hours spent in direct patient care or patient related service during the most recent complete week of practice by family physicians, May 2002. Available at: www.aafp.org/x769.xml.

[9] Hanley WB, Hanley AJG. The efficacy of stethoscope placement when not in use: traditional versus "cool." CMAJ 2000;163(12):1562–3.

[10] Minden, V. Improvement tip: do today's work today. Available at: www.ihi.org/resources/qi/qitips/ci0403tip.asp.

[11] Typical and acceptable waiting room waits. Available at: www.docrates.net/quickReport/typicalwait.htm.

[12] Does your opinion of your doctor change when you have to wait in the waiting room a long time? Available at: www.docrates.net/QuickReport/waitingroom.htm.

[13] Marvel MK, Epstein RM, Flowers K, Beckman HB. Soliciting the patient's agenda: have we improved? JAMA 1999;281(3):283–7.

[14] Bean RB, Bean WB, editors. Sir William Osler: Aphorisms from his bedside teaching and writings, II. The ethos. Available at: www.vh.org/adult/provider/history/osler/2.html. Accessed October 3, 2003.

[15] Flocke SA, Frank SH, Wenger DA. Addressing multiple problems in the family practice office visit. J Fam Pract 2001;50(3):211–6.

[16] Vincent C. Understanding and responding to adverse events. N Engl J Med 2003; 348(11):1051.

[17] Nease DE, Green LA. Clinfotracker: a generalizable prompting tool for primary care. J Fam Pract 2003;16(2):115–23.

[18] Flocke SA, Goodwin MA, Stange KC. The effect of the secondary patient on the family practice visit. J Fam Pract 1998;46(5):429–34.

[19] Houck S, Kilo C, Scott JC. Group visits 101. Family Practice Management 2003;10(5): 66–70.

[20] Thoesen Coleman M, Endsley S. Quality improvement: first steps. Family Practice Management 1999;6(5):23–44.

[21] Schwarz M, Landis SE, Row JE. A team approach to quality improvement. Family Practice Management 1999;6(4):25–32.

[22] Giovina JM. Holding the gains in quality improvement. Family Practice Management 1999;6(5):29–34.

[23] Zazove P, Klinkman M. Developing a CQI program in a family medicine department. Journal of Quality Improvement 1998;24(8):391–406.

Address reprint requests to

Randall T. Forsch, MD, MPH
Chelsea Family Practice Center
14700 E. Old US 12
Chelsea, MI 48118-0738

e-mail: rforsch@umich.edu

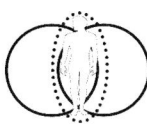 PROFESSIONAL AND PRACTICE MANAGEMENT SKILLS 1522–5720/03 $15.00 + .00

INTEGRATING INFORMATION TECHNOLOGY INTO CLINICAL PRACTICE

Mark H. Ebell, MD, MS

I do not fear computers. I fear the lack of them.
— Isaac Asimov, author and scientist (1920–1992)

What business are you in? Ask a group of physicians that question and you are likely to hear answers such as:

The business of seeing patients.
The business of treating disease.
The business of delivering health care.
The business of keeping my patients happy and paying the bills.

Although all of the above are true to some extent, they also miss the big picture. You may not know it, but you are really in the information business. As a physician, you first gather information from your patients when you interview and examine them, and combine it with what you know about the patient's medical history, their values, their community, and their family. Next, you integrate it with your personal medical knowledge base, which is, in turn, modified and informed by your clinical experience. Next, you formulate a treatment plan or course of action and communicate that back to your patient, the laboratory, colleagues, consultants, and the payor. You then record that information in the patient's medical record, adding to their "data warehouse."

A model of the flow of information during a typical patient encounter is shown in Fig. 1. The typical primary care physician has a panel of over 2000 patients and participates in 5000 or more patient encounters per year. Most patient encounters generate one or more clinical questions, although

Associate Professor, Department of Family Practice, Michigan State University, East Lansing, Michigan
The author is also co-founder of InfoPOEMs and author of the InfoRetriever software program.

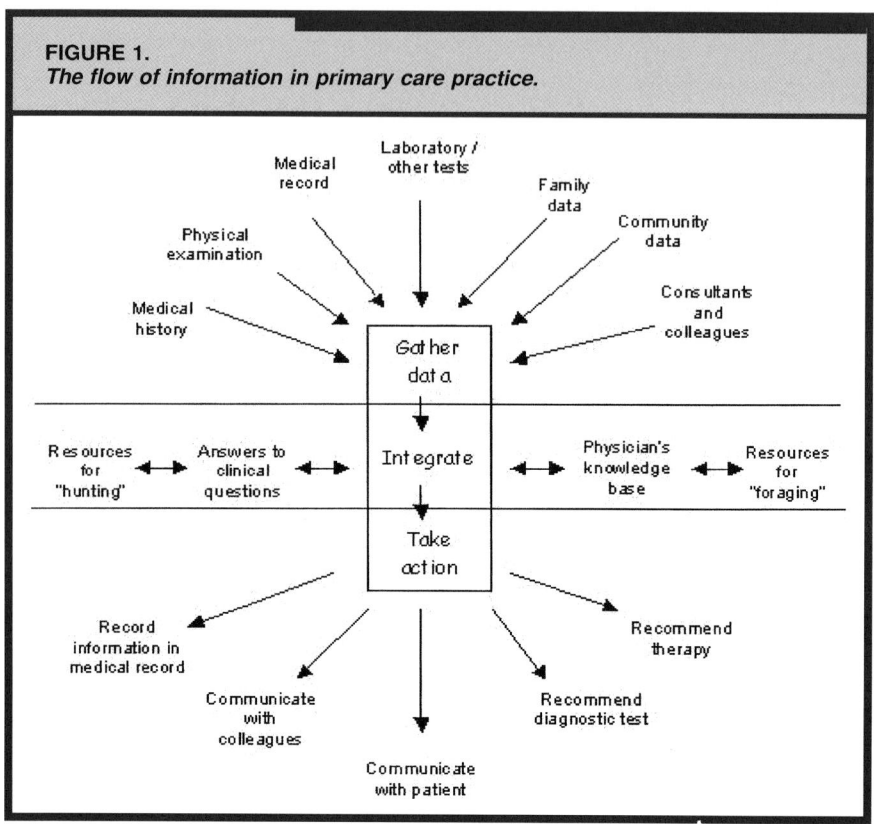

FIGURE 1.
The flow of information in primary care practice.

the bulk of these thousands of questions per year currently go unanswered [1–4]. The top 100 English-language clinical medical journals publish over 16,000 original research articles per year; a physician would have to read one ever 5 minutes for 220 ten-hour days to get through them all.

Clearly, clinicians are drowning in a sea of information, and the water is getting deeper; most physicians still use old or even ancient tools to manage information. Consider when each of the following was developed:

- Paper→105 ad
- Telephone→1876
- Problem-oriented medical record→1960s
- Fax machine→1843, widespread use 1970s

The average auto mechanic, overnight mail delivery person, and cash register operator uses more information technology in their workplaces than do 90% of American physicians. The average Starbuck's coffee shop has a wireless network, and you can walk into any Saturn dealer in the country and get your car's complete automotive history. Clearly, we can do better. Increasing attention is being paid to medical errors in the outpatient setting, and is forcing a re-evaluation of traditional systems for managing information. Sticky notes, illegible prescriptions, poor communication, incomplete documentation, and mangled dictation tapes will not be acceptable forever.

This article explores how information technology can help physicians to master the flow of information in their offices. Information technology includes hardware (computer equipment), software (computer programs that tell the hardware what to do), and wetware (the thoughts and ideas in the brain that provide an organizing framework for how to use information). All three are discussed in this article.

WETWARE

In Fig. 1, there are two branches at the integration step. The first branch, to the right, occurs when physicians access their personal "knowledge base." That knowledge base was stocked during training, and must be restocked continuously throughout physicians' careers. The second branch, to the left, indicates those times when the knowledge base is insufficient and physicians have a clinical question. Shaughnessy et al [5] call these two information needs "foraging" and "hunting," and have developed a framework called "Information Mastery" to help clinicians meet those information needs with the best available evidence.

Foraging

Physicians' medical knowledge base should be kept up to date with new information, but all too often it is not. In fact, in one survey, the best predictor of a physician's knowledge about hypertension was his or her year of graduation from medical school. Board scores typically show a steady decline the longer a physician has been out of school [6]. Although some of this may be due to an erosion of test-taking skills and greater specialization, it is not a reassuring trend.

Given the number of journals and research articles, physicians need a framework for identifying the most useful information. Shaughnessy et al [5] propose that the usefulness of information is related to relevance (how well the information applies to your patients and practice), validity (the strength of the evidence), and work (the effort needed to access information) in the following way:

$$\text{Usefulness of medical information} = \frac{\text{Relevance} \times \text{Validity}}{\text{Work}}$$

The most useful information, therefore, is highly relevant, of excellent validity, and takes very little effort to access. So what is relevant? Research that studies a common or important problem in a practice, measures patient-oriented outcomes rather than surrogate disease endpoints, and has the potential to change practice is the most relevant, and is called "patient-oriented evidence that matters" (POEM) [5].

Validity is determined by applying well-accepted principles of clinical epidemiology and research design. However, this is a lot of work, and requires training in biostatistics and epidemiology that most physicians do not have. To reduce work, Slawson and Shaughnessy [5] recommend that clinicians rely on others to do an initial screen for relevance, assess the validity, and summarize it for them. Examples of such information sources include POEMs (www.infopoems.com), ACP Journal Club (www.acp.org), and Clinical Evidence (www.clinicalevidence.com).

Because physicians spend only 2 to 8 hours per month reading to keep up with the literature [6], it makes sense that they make the best possible use of this time. Wading through original research articles in the *New England Journal of Medicine*, relying on chance or whatever catches their eye to determine relevance, and reviewing only journals to which they subscribe are inefficient and ineffective methods. Instead, physicians should subscribe to a medical information service that does the work for them.

Hunting

Foraging is only part of the answer to navigating the medical information jungle. We carnivores must be able to hunt as well! In this context, hunting means generating a clinical question, answering it with the best available evidence at the point of care, and applying it to the care of a patient. This process is shown in Fig. 2.

Perhaps the most important point in this pathway is the first step—that sense of unease, discomfort, or even downright ignorance that causes the physician to ask a clinical question. Although personal attributes such as curiosity and conscientiousness probably play a role, traditional continuing medical education and information services such as those described above also can serve an important role by making clinicians aware of new tests and treatments.

It's not enough to just ask a question. Physicians need the following basic "information mastery" skills:

Framing (restating) a question in a way that makes it easier to answer
Familiarity with sources of evidence-based information
Computer and searching skills
An understanding of the basic principles of evidence-based medicine

Physicians also need time. Fortunately, there are now tools available that bring large databases of evidence-based information to handheld computers (such as Clinical Evidence and InfoRetriever) and high-speed Internet connections that are always on. By not having to walk down the hall or dial up the Internet, physicians are able to answer questions faster and easier.

FIGURE 2.
The information pathway: asking and answering clinical questions.

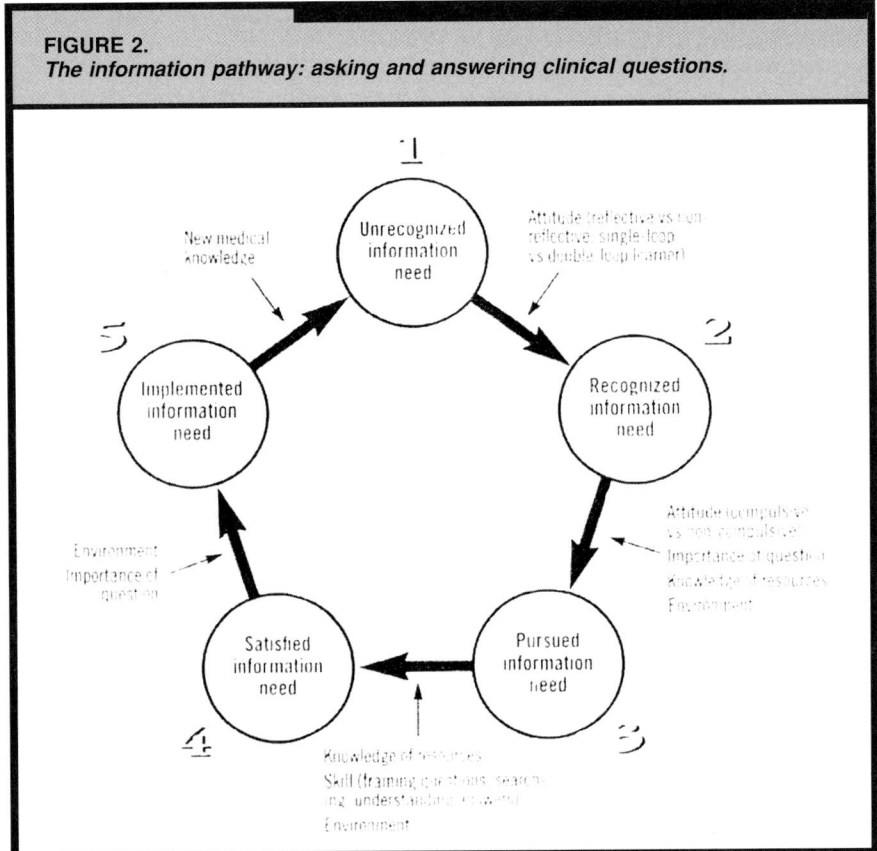

Systems

An important wetware principle is that you should try to build quality into the care process wherever possible. Make it hard to do the wrong thing, and easy to do the right thing. For example, most family physicians admit patients to the hospital with one of several common diagnoses (chest pain, pneumonia, congestive heart failure, chronic obstructive pulmonary disease, and asthma) on a regular basis. Rather than reinventing the wheel each time, develop a set of preprinted orders that help you translate evidence-based guidelines into practice. This can be done by an individual, a group practice, or even a medical staff. You do not need hardware and software to implement this concept, improve the quality of care, and reduce inappropriate variation in care.

Another simple wetware concept is flow charts and standardized templates for common outpatient problems. A sample encounter form for patients with sore throat is shown in Fig. 3; it is based on a validated

FIGURE 3.
Sore throat encounter form.

Figure 3. Sore Throat Encounter Form
Patient Name: _____ Medical Record #: _____ Age: _____

Data collection
☐ Palatine petchiae or scarlatinaform rash -> PROBABLE STREP

Symptom	Pts
☐ Fever	1
☐ Absence of cough	1
☐ Cervical adenopathy	1
☐ Tonsillar exudate	1
Age	
☐ < 15 years	+ 1
☐ 15-45 years	0
☐ > 45 years	-1
Total:	

Consider strep if:
☐ Contact with strep last 2 wks
☐ Duration of illness < 3 days

Consider mononucleosis if:
☐ Posterior cervical adenopathy

Consider abscess if:
☐ Hot-potato voice
☐ Sudden/severe symptoms

Consider meningitis if:
☐ Headache ☐ Stiff neck

0 / –1 points: strep ruled out (2%)
1-3 points: order rapid test and treat accordingly
4-5 points: probable strep (52%); consider empiric antibiotics

Rapid strep test: ___ Pos ___ Neg ___ NA   Mono spot: ___ Pos ___ Neg ___ NA
Other history:
_____
_____

Treatment
☐ Probable or confirmed strep pharyngitis
     Pen VK _____
     Cephalexin _____
     Erythromycin _____
     Azithromax _____

     Other: _____

☐ Viral pharyngitis   ☐ Mononucleosis
☐ Other _____

Symptomatic measures
     ☐ NSAIDs   ☐ 2% lidocaine gargle
     ☐ Chloraseptic   ☐ Salt water gargles

Other treatment: _____

clinical decision rule, and has the potential to speed documentation and improve the quality and consistency of care.

HARDWARE

If the automobile had followed the same development cycle as the computer, a Rolls-Royce would today cost $100, get a million miles per gallon, and explode once a year, killing everyone inside.
—Robert X. Cringely, *InfoWorld* magazine

Computer hardware has gotten cheaper, smaller, and faster at an incredible pace. The most important consequence of this for physicians is that they now can have access to information in their office, at home, in the hospital, at the nursing home, and even while watching their child's soccer game. This section briefly describes key technologies and their implications for family physicians. Table 1 summarizes the key recommendations for equipping an office.

TABLE 1.
Hardware Recommendations

Item	Price Range	Recommendation
Desktop computers	$400 to $1000	• Flat panel 15″ or larger monitor to save space • 30 GB hard drive • Built-in network card • 256 MB random access memory
Laptop computer	$800 to $2000	• As above for desktop computer 1except XGA or SXGA screen • If you plan to travel a lot, keep the weight under 4 pounds and battery life over 4 hours
Broadband access (residential)	$40 to $60	• Begin with the midrange download speed
Broadband access (business)	$200 to $500	• Service guarantee • 24/7 on-site service
Tablet computer	$1500 to $2500	• At least a 4-hour battery life • Weight under 4 pounds, ideally under 3 • Extra battery and battery charger
Handheld computer	$100 to $600	• Size—if you want to carry it in your shirtpocket, will it fit comfortably? • Internal memory: 8–16 MB for Palm, 64 MB or more for Pocket PC • At least one and preferably two storage card slots • View screen indoors and out • Processor—400 MHz X-Scale for Pocket PC, 140 MHz ARM or higher for Palm • Consider built-in wifi or integration with cell phone

Broadband Connectivity

The term bandwidth refers to the size of the "pipe" that connects a computer to the Internet. A "broadband" connection is a big pipe that can send data quickly from the Internet to a computer and from a computer back to the Internet. The most common types of broadband connections are cable modems and digital subscriber lines (DSL). Usually, it is possible to choose from a menu of download speeds, from approximately 256 kilobytes per second to over 1000 kps (compared with a typical effective speed of 28 to 40 kps for dial-up service). The price of 1 month of service is typically $35 to $50.

There are differences between cable modems and DSL connections. With a cable modem, the connection to the Internet is shared through a hub in a specific region, so if there are more people online, speed suffers. Most vendors offer a minimum speed guarantee, however. DSL lines offer a more consistent download speed, but may be more affected by local electrical interference. Reliability is especially important when an Application Service Provider (ASP) model is used for electronic medical records (EMRs; ie, data are stored in a separate location and accessed through the Internet). In that case, it may be worth paying more per month (typically $200 to $500 per month) for a more reliable connection with a service guarantee.

Even if an ASP is not used for EMRs, there are many reasons why a broadband connection should be considered. First, not only are broadband connections fast, but, perhaps even more importantly, they are always on. Instead of waiting an interminable minute or two while the computer whistles and squeaks to connect over a phone line, with broadband, it is possible to just walk up to the computer and start accessing information. Online references are suddenly a valuable resource, and you can start to retire some of your textbooks. The cost is partially offset by not having to have a phone line. Plus, if all the computers in an office are networked, the same high-speed Internet connection can be shared.

Networks can be wired or wireless. Wireless networks are now just as fast and much more convenient than are wired networks, because they do not limit a computer to one location in each room, and do not require holes being dug in the walls to lay cable. If a wireless network is installed, however, it is still necessary to configure it to comply with Health Insurance Portability and Accountability Act security standards. This should be done by an experienced computer network technician—most practices would benefit from finding such a person or company locally to install and maintain their network.

Tablet or Slate Computers

For many years, a number of companies have made "tablet" computers, which resemble an Etch-a-Sketch, weigh about 3 or 4 pounds, and do not have a built-in keyboard. Recently, Microsoft (Redmond, Washington) created a special version of its Microsoft Windows operating system for "Tablet PCs," and created a set of specifications for this type of computer (http://www.microsoft.com/windowsxp/tabletpc/default.asp). Most now have a screen that twists on its axis so they can behave like a normal laptop or like a slate.

Tablet PCs are well suited to the medical workplace. The screen is much larger than that of a handheld computer, and they can run any software that runs on your desktop computer. Most have wireless networking built in; thus, information can be shared constantly with the office's server (the main storage computer in a network) or even with the Internet. The form factor is similar to what physicians are used to—writing on an $8'' \times 11''$ flat surface. Software is adapted to minimize the amount of typing needed—in most cases you check a box or select from a list. The two major drawbacks compared with handheld computers are the battery life and weight. Three or four pounds does not sound like much until you lug it around for 10 hours! The battery life should be adequate to allow you to work all day, plugging into an electrical socket only overnight and during the lunch hour. Most devices currently have a 3- to 4-hour battery life, so an extra battery is a necessity for the busy clinician.

Handheld Computers

> Where a calculator on the ENIAC is equipped with 18,000 vacuum tubes and weighs 30 tons, computers in the future may have only 1000 vacuum tubes and perhaps weigh 1.5 tons.
>
> —Unknown, *Popular Mechanics*, March 1949

If you stop by a medical school, you'll see that almost every student has a handheld computer. The vast majority of residents also have one, although older physicians have been somewhat slower to adopt these devices. As a clinician you are in the information business; therefore, it makes sense to have access to that information wherever you go.

One hurdle that keeps many physicians from purchasing a handheld computer is "analysis paralysis." They keep waiting for the next great handheld computer to be developed, and end up never buying one. (This can happen with other kinds of computer technology as well.) Get over it! Yes, next year's model will be a bit faster and have new features, but if you purchase a handheld computer today for $200 to $400, it will give you at least 2 to 3 years of solid service.

When your personal digital assistant starts to show its age, you usually can upgrade the operating system for little or no cost. This is because the operating system (the basic instructions that control the computer's operations) on many handheld computers is stored in "flash memory" and can be upgraded after downloading an update from the manufacturer's Web site. Because memory cards are cheap, it also is possible to add more memory to an older device; a 256-megabyte (MB) storage card costs between $25 and $50 depending on the type of card. That size of card can hold dozens of medical references, 60 songs in MP3 format, or even an entire movie!

Which operating system (OS) should you choose, Palm or Pocket PC? The conventional wisdom held that the Palm OS was cheaper and easier to use, whereas the Pocket PC was more powerful and had a larger screen, but also was more expensive and harder to master. This has changed recently, and it is now possible to purchase a Pocket PC for about $200, whereas the latest device that runs the Palm operating system can cost over $400.

There are some clear differences between handheld computers running the Palm and Pocket PC operating systems. Palm devices usually have more software (although this is changing quickly) and a somewhat more intuitive user interface. Although the battery life is somewhat better, this difference is not as pronounced as it once was because most of the Palm OS devices have gotten larger, more power-hungry color screens like their Pocket PC brethren.

Pocket PCs offer faster, more powerful processors and higher screen resolutions than do most Palm OS devices, as well as built-in audio and color in every device, better wireless capability, and increased security features (ie, encryption for wireless). Both devices offer some degree of integration with Microsoft Word and Excel, although the Pocket PC offers better integration with Outlook out of the box.

It is worth visiting your local electronics or office supply store to take a look at the screen of the models that you are considering before you buy. Do not forget to take a look at the screen outdoors in bright light if you plan to use it on the golf course!

Make sure you get plenty of built-in storage memory—at least 8 to 16 MB for the Palm OS device, and 32 MB to 64 MB for the Pocket PC (Pocket PC programs are larger and less efficient at using memory than are Palm OS programs). Your device also should have at least one, and ideally two, slots for storage cards; you can keep dozens of medical applications on one card, music on another, and recorded books on a third. Having an expansion slot also lets you connect to a network or even the Internet with a wireless or wired modem. In my home, I have a cable modem that connects to a "router," and wireless network cards for each laptop and for my Pocket PC. The entire setup cost less than $300, and allows me to connect to the Internet with a high-speed connection from my Pocket PC or laptop anywhere in my home. You can get help with selecting the correct equipment from a local electronics retailer such as Radio Shack—at a minimum, you will need a router with 802.11b connectivity (approximately $100) and an 802.11b compatible network card for each computer ($50 each) or handheld device ($70 to $100 each). Linksys Inc. (Irvine, California), Microsoft (Redmond, Washington), and other companies manufacture this hardware.

SOFTWARE

One way of describing software is that it is the set of instructions that allows your wetware (brain) to control your hardware. This section discusses software that supports four important tasks: EMR management, decision support and medical reference access, electronic prescribing, and patient education.

EMRs

Although over 95% of family physicians use computers at home, and the vast majority uses them to assist in billing and financial operations of their practice, less than 10% currently are using an EMR [7]. There are

TABLE 2.
Advantages and Disadvantages of an EMR

Advantages	Disadvantages
Available 24/7 to physician and to any partners or call coverage	Expensive
No issues with handwriting	Decreased productivity during learning curve
Reduced transcription costs	If computer or network fails, no access to records
Electronic prescribing reduces errors and pharmacy callbacks	
Enter data once, use it in many ways (progress note, letter to consultant, billing documentation)	
May improve coding and reduce medicolegal risk	

many arguments in favor of using an EMR, but these are balanced by important barriers [8], as shown in Table 2.

A number of important trends are shifting the balance in favor of using an EMR. These include:

> The increasing complexity of medical care, with more patients on multiple medications, and the consequent increase in the likelihood of errors of omission and commission
>
> An increasingly mobile population that requires more efficient information sharing between physicians
>
> Increasing computer literacy in the physician and patient populations
>
> Greater reporting requirements
>
> The need to provide audit trails for access to medical records
>
> Incentives from malpractice insurers and insurance companies for using electronic prescribing and EMRs

There are many obvious benefits to EMRs. They reduce or eliminate problems with poor handwriting; include electronic prescribing, which reduces medical errors and pharmacy callbacks; are available 24 hours a day; do not get lost; and can be used by several people at once [8]. They also reduce duplicate effort—on a typical visit, I will write a progress note, write some instructions for the patient, and dictate a letter to a consultant or colleague. I write a prescription, and then update the patient's medication list. With an EMR, data entered once can be used any number of times.

Perhaps most importantly, using an EMR gives physicians a way to systematically monitor and improve the quality of the care that they deliver. For example, when Baycol (cerivastatin) was removed from the market, physicians with an EMR could easily generate a list of their patients taking the mediation. It also is possible to generate reminders quickly, receive decision support regarding laboratory testing [9,10], identify patients who are not meeting their goals for blood sugar or blood pressure control, and tailor patient education to the patient's needs.

Most EMRs use a system of templates for different types of visits—a template for sore throat, a template for urinary tract infection, and a template for chest pain. This gives physicians another way to improve the quality and consistency of care, because they generally can modify these templates to reflect an evidence-based approach to care, which makes it easier to do the right thing for patients and harder to omit something or commit an error. In some cases, users have even banded together to share these templates. For example, Logician (an EMR from GE Medical Systems, Milwaukee, Wisconsin) has developed a KnowledgeBank that contains hundreds of templates from practices around the country, freely available for downloading (http://knowledge.medicalogic.com/index.jsp).

All of this power is not cheap, however. There is the cost of the EMR itself, the cost of integrating it with existing medical billing systems, and the lost productivity over the first 6 months or so as physicians get up to speed with the new system. These costs are balanced by cost savings—fewer chart pulls, fewer pharmacy callbacks, lower or eliminated dictation costs, lower or eliminated chart storage costs, charge capture improvement, billing error decrease, more efficient prescribing and laboratory use, and the possibility of greater workflow efficiency in the office. Studies of the financial impact of using an EMR are limited but encouraging [11–13], although the financial impact depends to some extent on the practice organization. Because many of the savings revolve around more cost-effective prescribing and diagnostic testing, these may be realized only in a staff model or heavily capitated managed care setting.

The most detailed and up-to-date cost analysis to date [13] estimated a cost per provider of $13,100 per year for the software, hardware, and support. This study also estimated a temporary productivity loss during the first 3 months of $11,200. The benefit was smallest for a minimal EMR implementation (online charts and electronic prescribing only) and greatest for a full EMR (charts, prescribing, laboratory and radiology order entry, and charge capture). The degree of benefit was most sensitive to five variables, with a greater benefit seen in the following settings:

Greater proportion of patients in capitated health plans
Drug savings benefit the practice
A lower discount rate for managed care patients
A larger panel size per physician
A greater degree of transcription reduction

A particularly bad combination was a low percentage of capitated patients and a high discount rate, with a net benefit over 5 years that was as low as $3000 per physician. On the other hand, practices with a high percentage of capitated patients that benefit from drug savings had a 5-year net benefit of over $200,000 per provider. Even in a worst-case analysis, using an EMR had a net cost of only $2300 per provider. Almost all other sets of assumptions showed a net financial benefit for using an EMR.

An excellent source of information about EMRs is the annual comparison published in *Family Practice Management* (www.aafp.org/fpm). The American Academy of Family Physicians, which publishes *Family Practice Management*, recently has announced an initiative to deliver a low-cost, primary-care-oriented EMR to its members within the next 2 to 3 years (http://www.aafp.org/x19017.xml). If they are successful, it could reduce greatly the cost and risk of adopting an EMR.

As you consider adoption of an EMR, review the Wang article [13] and think about where your practice falls on the spectrum of the five variables. Some important questions to ask as you shop for an EMR are as follows:

Do I want to use a mix of paper and EMR, or go completely paperless?

Does the vendor provide on-site support?

How much does support cost?

Does the EMR use an open database standard (good) or a proprietary database technology (bad)?

Does the user interface allow me to modify the data entry templates to fit my practice?

How well does the system handle visits for multiple problems, so common in the primary care setting?

How much will it cost to integrate this system into my existing practice management system?

Because many of the potential benefits of an EMR accrue to patients, payers, and the health system in general (more cost-effective prescribing, more cost-effective use of the laboratory, greater adherence to evidence-based practice guidelines, fewer medical errors), it is important that insurance companies and the federal government take a role in encouraging the use of EMRs, perhaps by providing enhanced reimbursement for physicians who use them [8].

Decision Support and Medical Reference Access

As discussed earlier, the "usefulness equation" [5] helps clinicians to understand that the most useful information is relevant, valid, and takes little work to access. However, physicians too often rely on sources of information that are out-of-date, take too long to access, or are not relevant to their patients or questions. Examples include an old textbook (be honest, what is the average age of textbooks on your office bookshelf?), a Medline search that yields thousands of "hits," a pharmaceutical representative who has the goal of promoting his or her product as well as providing information, and a colleague whose knowledge base is out-of-date. Too often, questions go unanswered because it is too much work, or are not answered with the best available information.

This section describes some useful sources of high-quality information, with an emphasis on evidence-based sources (see Table 3 for a

TABLE 3.
High-Quality and Evidence-Based Reference Sources

Source	Location
Evidence based	
InfoRetriever	http://www.infopoems.com
Clinical Evidence	http://www.clinicalevidence.org
Cochrane Library	http://www.update-software.com/cochrane/
ACP Journal Club	http://www.acpjc.org
Other key sources	
PubMed clinical queries	http://www.ncbi.nlm.nih.gov/entrez/query/static/clinical.html
TRIP database	http://www.tripdatabase.com
Dynamed	http://www.dynamicmedical.com

summary). What is an evidence-based source? The sine qua non is that the source explicitly rates the strength of evidence for key clinical recommendations. Although many sources describe themselves as evidence based, only those that rate the strength of evidence consistently deserve that label. It also is important to note how often information is updated, whether the source uses a systematic approach in evaluating relevance, and whether they make an effort to reduce a physician's work.

Some truly evidence-based sources include the Cochrane Library, InfoRetriever, Clinical Evidence, and the ACP Journal Club. InfoRetriever, which my colleagues and I have developed over the past 10 years, integrates a systematic literature surveillance built around over 2400 POEMs, abstracts from the Cochrane Database of Systematic Reviews, evidence-based guideline summaries from the National Guidelines Clearinghouse, an extensive database of diagnostic test information, over 120 clinical decision guides, the 5-Minute Clinical Consult, and an extensive medical photo database. It is designed around the usefulness equation: a single query searches all databases simultaneously, data are summarized and "predigested" to reduce work, every item is labeled with the strength of evidence, and the literature surveillance uses the "POEMs" criteria to ensure relevance. The database is available for the desktop computer, Palm OS, Pocket PC, and via a Web browser. Some sample screen shots are shown in Fig. 4.

Clinical Evidence is from the editors of the *British Medical Journal*, and provides concise, evidence-based summaries of common problems. Largely devoted to treatment issues, each set of recommendations is organized into groups according to the degree of benefit or harm: "Likely to be beneficial," "Unknown effectiveness," "Likely to be ineffective or harmful," and so on. It is updated twice a year and is an excellent source of evidence-based treatment information.

The Cochrane Library performs systematic reviews of key clinical topics, scouring the world's literature to identify all of the clinical trials on

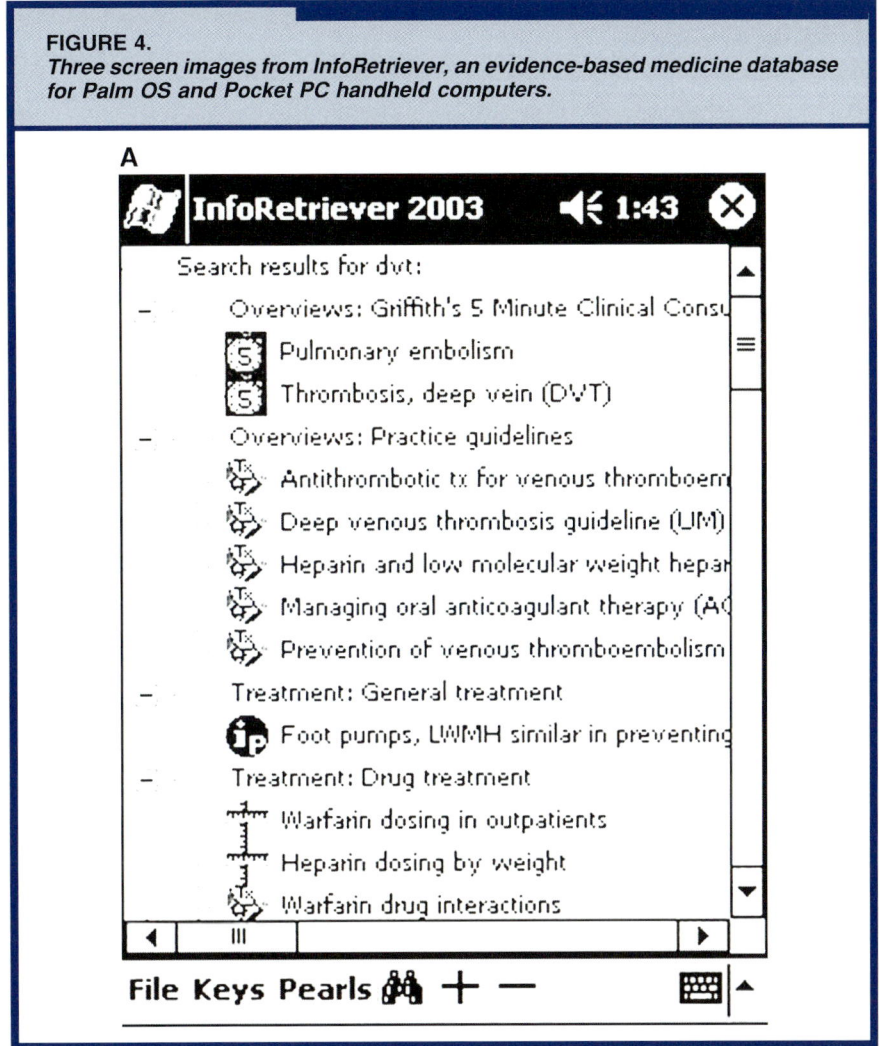

FIGURE 4.
Three screen images from InfoRetriever, an evidence-based medicine database for Palm OS and Pocket PC handheld computers.

a topic. They then evaluate the quality of the evidence, and—using a rigorous protocol—write a systematic review. There have been over 1600 reviews published to date, with another 3000 or so planned over the next 10 years. The Cochrane Library also includes other databases—in particular, a collection of over 300,000 abstracts of clinical trials, many of which are not found in Medline.

The ACP Journal Club is a subscription service from the American College of Physicians. Their reviewers perform regular literature surveillance, with an emphasis on adult medicine. Each summary includes an abstract and a clinical commentary.

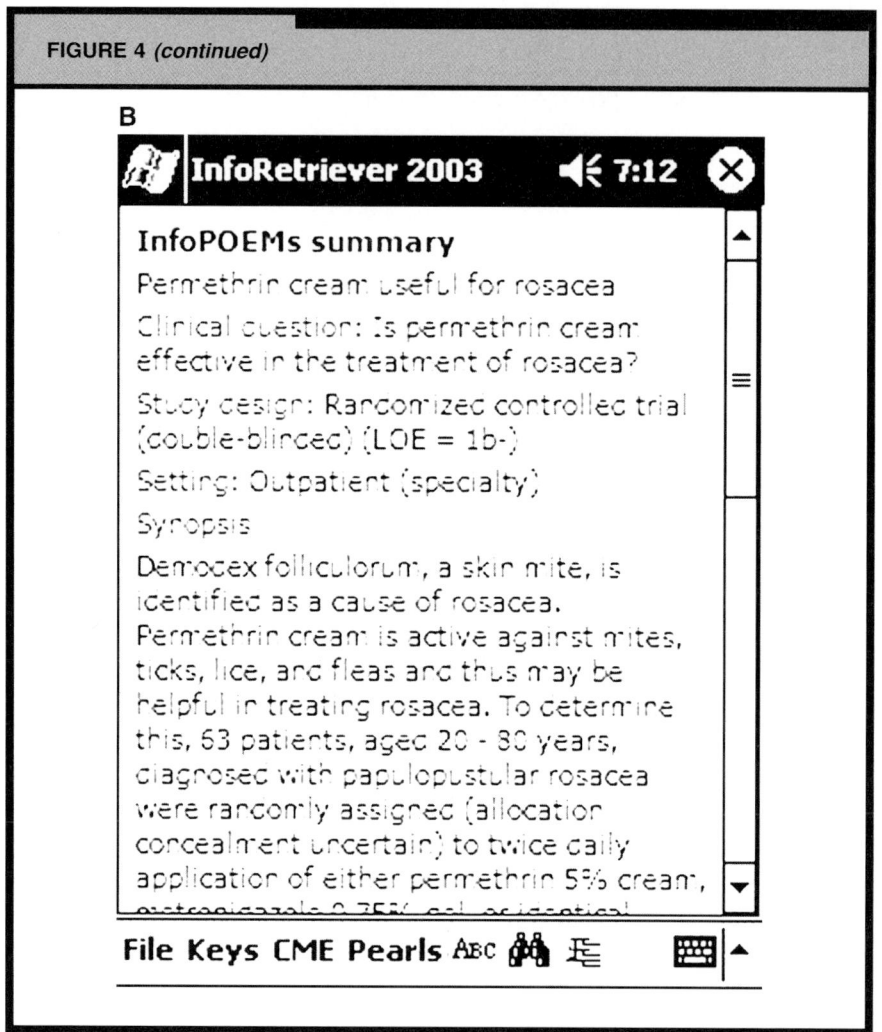

FIGURE 4 (continued)

PubMed is the well-known and widely used interface to Medline. Although more user friendly than in the past, the main PubMed search engine still can be a challenge, and requires considerable experience. An especially helpful hint for clinicians is to use the "Clinical queries" subpage, which can be accessed from a link on the site's main page (http://www.ncbi.nlm.nih.gov/entrez/query/static/clinical.html). This subpage allows you to enter a search term; indicate whether you are looking for information on diagnosis, prognosis, etiology, or treatment; and then indicate whether you want a sensitive (broad) or specific (narrow) search. The results are much more likely to be relevant than are those from a

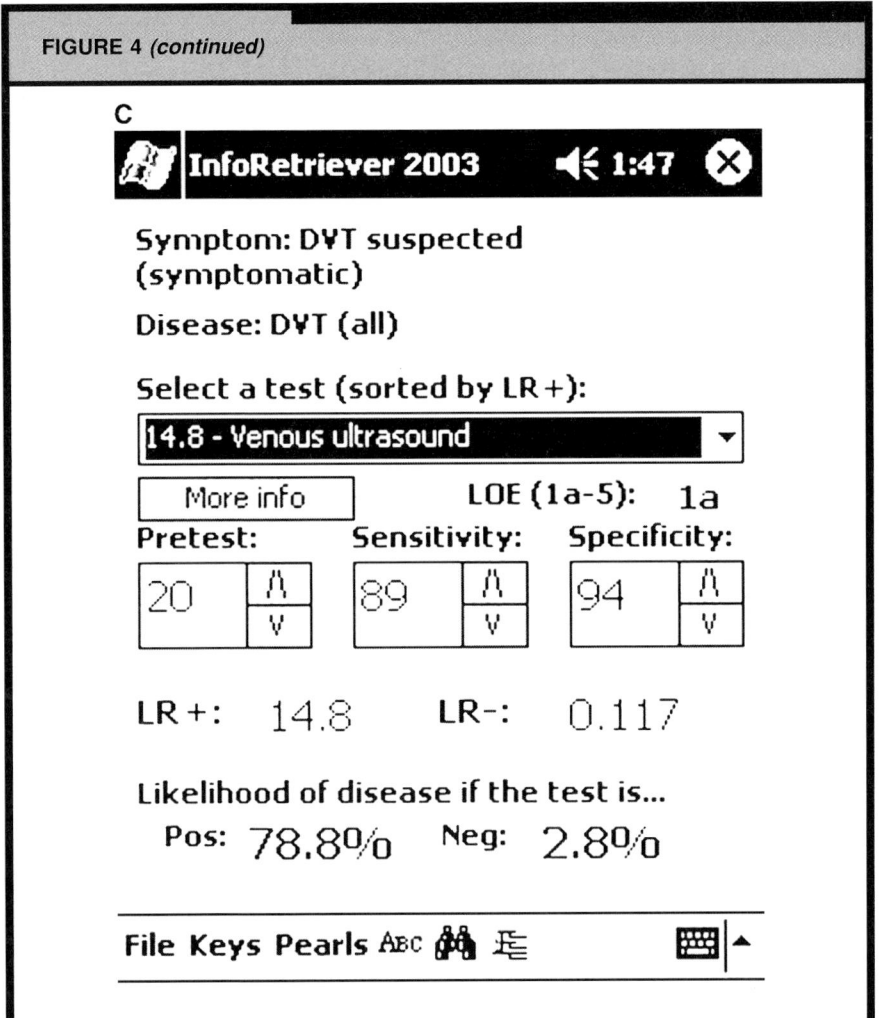

FIGURE 4 *(continued)*

traditional Medline search, but it still is more work than using a "predigested" source such as Clinical Evidence or InfoRetriever.

Another site that is not well known in the United States is TRIP: Translating Research Into Practice. This "meta-site" searches 75 other Web sites simultaneously, and specifically identifies evidence-based sites of information. The basic search is free, and you can subscribe to obtain more detailed search results. A sample search result for "deep vein thrombosis" is shown in Fig. 5.

DynaMed is a site developed by Brian Alper, MD, and currently contains over 1600 topics. Although it does not label explicitly the strength

FIGURE 5.
TRIP database screen shot. From *www.tripdatabase.com; with permission.*

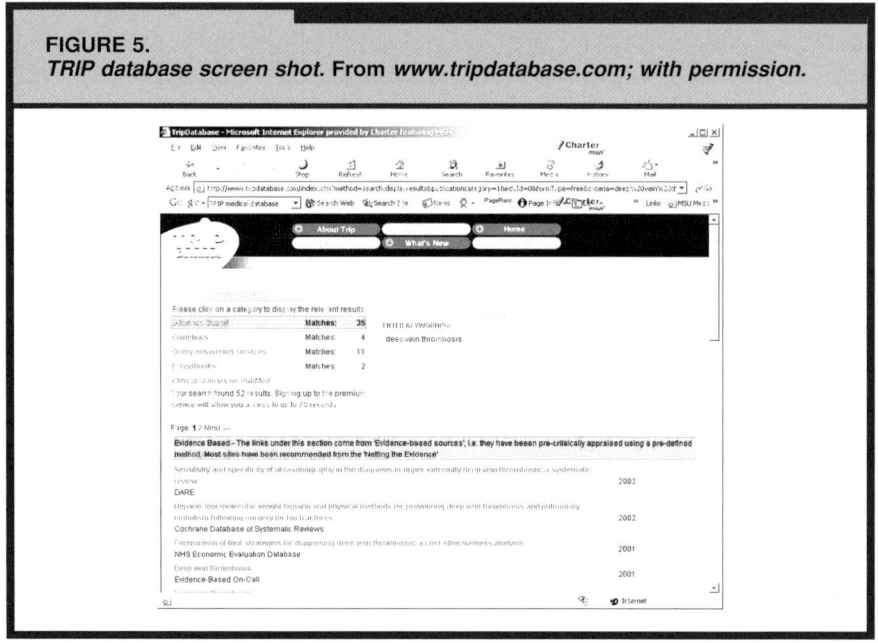

of evidence, it does provide considerable information about study design and has an "EBM feel" to it. Previously free, the site is moving to a subscription model and beginning the process of peer reviewing the topics.

Electronic Prescribing and Patient Education

Electronic prescribing and patient education usually are built into EMRs. However, it also is possible to obtain them in stand-alone products, which is a nice way for physicians to dip their toes into the water of clinical informatics. Examples of patient education software include Medifor (http://publishing.allscripts.com/products/fs2.html, Chicago, Illinois) and Clinical Reference Systems (http://publishing.allscripts.com/products/fs2.html, Chicago, Illinois). Over 500 patient education topics also can be viewed at and printed from the free site sponsored by the American Academy of Family Physicians (http://www.familydoctor.org), which even includes translations into Spanish for many documents. InfoRetriever, described above, includes indexed links to all of these topics for users of their software who have Internet access.

Electronic prescribing has migrated largely to handheld computers, often using wireless networks to send prescriptions to a printer or even directly to the pharmacy. Handheld computers can reduce time needed for callbacks; time wasted writing and rewriting prescriptions ("Oh by the way, can you rewrite those 12 prescriptions for my mail-in pharmacy"?);

medical errors caused by handwriting; and, with integrated interaction checking, can reduce other kinds of medical errors as well. Vendors include AllScripts (www.allscripts.com, Chicago, Illinois), PocketScript (www.pocketscript.com, Mason, Ohio), iScribe (www.iscribe.com, Irving, Texas), and Bluefish RX (www.bluefishrx.com, San Francisco, California). All but iScribe, which uses the Palm, use the Pocket PC platform. Electronic prescribing can be an excellent way to introduce your staff to the benefits of computers in the clinical workplace, while improving the quality of care that you deliver to your patients.

SUMMARY

Hopefully, this article has given you some ideas for your practice. Why don't you make a list right now of three things that you plan to adopt in your practice—for example, subscribe to an information service, contact at least three electronic prescribing vendors for estimates, and get broadband access for the computers in your clinic. Begin to place more value on the questions that you ask in your practice and answer important ones with the best available evidence. Talk to your partners about the pros and cons of an EMR. The journal *Family Practice Management* has a terrific toolkit that includes calculators and spreadsheets for helping you make this decision, as well as lots of charting tools to make your practice more systematic (http://www.aafp.org/x20091.xml). Time to get started!

Key Points

- Physicians have two types of information needs: foraging to keep up to date and hunting for answers to clinical questions.
- Information Mastery and POEMs is a framework that helps physicians find the most useful information: it is highly relevant, of excellent validity, and takes little effort to access.
- Key new technologies that can improve access to medical information are broadband connectivity, handheld computers, and wireless networks.
- A variety of factors are making EMRs a more attractive option for clinicians.
- The degree of financial benefit from an EMR is influenced most strongly by five variables: greater proportion of patients in capitated health plans, a drug-savings benefit to the practice for economic prescribing, a lower discount rate for managed care patients, a larger panel size per physician, and a greater degree of transcription reduction.
- Useful evidence-based electronic sources of information include the Cochrane Library, TRIP, InfoRetriever, and the ACP Journal Club.

References

[1] Ebell MH. Information at the point of care: answering clinical questions. J Am Board Fam Pract 1999;12(3):225–35.

[2] Covell DG, Uman GC, Manning PR. Information needs in office practice: are they being met? Ann Intern Med 1985;103:596–9.

[3] Smith R. What clinical information do doctors need? BMJ 1996;313:1062–8.

[4] Gorman PN, Helfand M. Information seeking in primary care: how physicians choose which clinical questions to pursue and which to leave unanswered. Med Decis Making 1995;15:113–9.

[5] Shaughnessy AF, Slawson DC, Bennett JH. Becoming an information master: a guidebook to the medical information jungle. J Fam Pract 1994;39(5):489–99.

[6] Sackett DL, Richardson WS, Rosenberg W, Haynes RB. Evidence-based medicine: how to practice and teach EBM. 1st edition. New York: Churchill-Livingstone; 1997. p. 8–9.

[7] Anderson JD. Increasing the acceptance of clinical information systems. MD Computing 1999;16:62–5.

[8] Bates DW, Ebell M, Gotlieb E, Zapp J, Mullins HC. A proposal for electronic medical records in US primary care. J Am Med Inform Assoc 2003;10:1–10.

[9] Tierney WM, Miller ME, McDonald CJ. The effect on test ordering of informing physicians of the charges for outpatient diagnostic tests. N Engl J Med 1990;322:1499–504.

[10] Tierney WM, McDonald CJ, Martin DK, Rogers MP. Computerized display of past test results. Effect on outpatient testing. Ann Intern Med 1987;107:549–74.

[11] Schmitt KF, Wofford DA. Financial analysis projects clear returns from electronic medical records. Healthcare Financial Management 2002;56(1):52–7.

[12] Renner K. Cost-justifying electronic medical records. Healthcare Financial Management 1996;50:63–4.

[13] Wang SJ, Middleton B, Prosser LA, et al. A cost–benefit analysis of electronic medical records in primary care. Am J Med 2003;114(5):397–403.

Address reprint requests to

Mark H. Ebell, MD, MS
330 Snapfinger Drive
Athens, GA 30605

e-mail: ebell@msu.edu

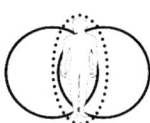
PROFESSIONAL AND PRACTICE MANAGEMENT SKILLS 1522–5720/03 $15.00 + .00

CLINIC SCHEDULING AND ACCESS

Philip Zazove, MD, MM

"You have an urgent message on your desk," my secretary told me as I entered my office. I walked to the desk and looked at the note. It was a message from a patient, complaining about the long wait time to see a doctor at one of my sites. This was the third complaint about physician access that week alone, not to mention the complaints I had received via telephone with regard to the long wait times. I knew full well that this was a problem many physicians and medical centers were facing all over the country; however, that knowledge did not make me feel any better. Patients have the right to expect prompt service, especially when they are not feeling well. I sighed and reached for the phone.

Access. It's a word that physicians are hearing regularly these days. Inadequate access to care is common [1,2], costly [3], and a major cause of low patient satisfaction, with approximately 25% of patients reporting dissatisfaction with "access to care" [4–8]. However, the term "access" means different things to different people [9]. To hospital administrators, it means increasing the effective number of beds, whether by building more space, adding new beds, or increasing throughput. To the forty million Americans without health insurance, it means coming up with the funds to afford to see a physician or obtain a needed procedure. To an increasing number of physicians—both primary care physicians and specialists—it means figuring out how to see all the patients who want to be seen on a timely basis, while providing high-quality medical care.

This article focuses on the last scenario, and looks at access from the perspective of a family practice physician's office. There is no universally agreed upon time frame for time frames for visit access wait times. Box 1 shows the parameters used by the University of Michigan's Faculty Group Practice for their primary care physicians. Other places have different parameters, however, and therefore it may be that the best time frame is what the patient thinks is reasonable.

From the Department of Family Medicine, University of Michigan, Ann Arbor, and Ambulatory Care Services, University of Michigan Hospitals and Health Centers, Dexter, Michigan

---

Box 1. Family Group Practice Access Standards for Primary Care

1. 100% of Primary Care Providers (PCPs) will be open to accept new patients. Patients may be offered another provider within the same health center for those PCPs who have panels that are filled.
2. Scheduled appointments for each health center will be available within:

- 30 days for nonsymptomatic office visits (ie, well-child, Health Maintenance Examination [HME])
- 2 weeks for first prenatal visit with provider
- 3 days for symptomatic office visits (ie, nonurgent)
- 24 hours for urgent visit

3. To extend appointment availability, provider hours will include nontraditional hours. Full full-time equivalent (FTE) staff members are expected to work 12 nontraditional hours per month (Family Practice, General Internal Medicine, Pediatrics), 9 nontraditional hours per month (Obstetrics/Gynecology). Nontraditional hours are defined as those hours other than Monday through Friday, 8:00 AM to 5:00 PM.
4. At least 6 weeks' advance notice will be given for anticipated provider clinic cancellations (ie, vacation, continuing medical education)

The continuing reductions in reimbursement for medical services coupled with the increasing demand of the population for medical care (due to technologic advances and the aging of America, among other reasons) is making it necessary to maximize the number of patients that can be seen. Moreover, service is one of the few ways in which practices can distinguish themselves in the marketplace [10]. Unfortunately, in many situations, this is not achieved easily; it is influenced by numerous variables, many of which interact.

DEFINITION

As stated previously, this article discusses access from the perspective of how family physicians can meet patient demand for quality care. Not surprisingly, coming up with a definition of access is not that simple. For example, the type of practice has significant implications for how access is addressed. A small, rural practice with only one or two doctors is a totally different situation than a large, urban, multiphysician academic practice. In the former case, the physicians may be the only doctors in the area and obligated to cover not only the emergency room and hospital patients, but also community-based health issues such as supervising emergency medical technicians and caring for local industry. This heavy load can restrict physicians' abilities to adhere to their schedule and can limit their hours. On the contrary, faculty in an urban medical school may only see patients a few days a week, due to teaching and research obligations, and while in the office, they may have medical students or residents with them every time they see a patient. This scenario creates totally different constraints with regard to the ability to see patients and other parameters such as continuity of care.

Similarly, other factors can influence which interventions to improve access may work at a particular practice, including ownership (private versus corporate versus academic), number and type of specialties at the site, competition in the community, and commitment of the physicians.

The above notwithstanding, the basic premise this article follows is that access can be increased best by "doing today's work today." Under this concept, access can be defined as patients receiving the care and information they need, when they need it [11,12]. The extent, to which this is accomplished, of course, depends on the specific practice variables enumerated earlier. This article discusses a variety of methods that physicians can implement to improve access. Each physician will need to decide which ones may apply to his or her unique situation.

INITIAL CONTACT WITH THE OFFICE

Many management consultants talk about the "moments of truth." These are the specific times in the interaction between customers and a business that are essential to providing a good impression so that the patient ends up at that business. In the medical office business, one such "moment of truth" is the initial contact the patient has with the office. Traditionally, this has been via the telephone, although increasingly it also is via the Internet. In addition to being key factors in creating the patient's first impression of the office, the telephone and Web site can play essential roles in impacting patient access.

Let's begin with the telephone. Imagine you woke up this morning with a pain in your left chest. You've had this multiple times before, but have put off talking to your doctor about it. Today, though, you become more worried than usual (after all, all your grandparents and one of your parents died of ateriosclerotic heart disease) because one of your staff was just hospitalized with unstable angina. You take an aspirin, move around, and try some food, but the pain persists. So you decide to call your doctor. You remember her office opens at 8 AM and look at your watch—it is 8:05. You pick up the phone and call.

After three rings, an automated voice answers and tells you that all lines are busy, to be patient, and that your call will be answered in the order in which it was received. Ten minutes later you're still hearing the voice tell you to be patient. You're having a hard time doing this, as the pain persists and you worry it may be your heart. At 15 minutes, when you are debating whether to hang up and go to the emergency room (knowing full well you'll probably wait a long time there too), someone finally answers.

It then takes another 10 minutes to make the appointment. First, you have to wait while they pull up your name in the computer, then scan the doctor's schedule to see when her next available appointment is. Then the staff member puts you on hold while she checks someone out. When she returns, it turns out that the doctor's schedule is full and they need to check if they can double-book her. It takes 5 minutes to get that approval, and another 5 minutes to update them with your new phone number and insurance. The entire time from when you dialed the number to hanging up—well over 25 minutes.

Now, imagine this scenario. You get the chest pain and decide to see your physician. You call her office, and on the second ring a live voice answers. She connects you with the appointment scheduler who, after a brief discussion of the available times, books you for 11:00 that morning. Then she updates your demographic and insurance information before you are finished. The entire time on the phone—8 minutes. In addition, the employee who makes the appointments now has time to help out with other office tasks while waiting for the next call.

Finally, how about this scenario. You get the chest pain and decide to make an appointment with your doctor. You get on your computer, click on the bookmark for her office, and make the appointment directly without speaking to anyone—total time, 90 seconds.

The impression of the office that a patient would get from each of these scenarios—an impression that is developed even before seeing the doctor—is obvious. Therefore, managing the telephones well is critical to a positive impression and a well-run practice. There are numerous issues to consider in the aim of creating efficient telephone interactions, including whether to have a live person or an automated attendant answer the phone initially; the use of call centers; appropriate staffing levels; and whether the practice should have a nurse or other person who can provide triage and other advice, and perform other duties [1,9]. It also helps to know the most common reasons for which patients in a particular practice call (eg, for an appointment, a prescription refill, a referral request, or to talk to the nurse) [13].

If possible, a telephone call analysis should be conducted to provide extensive information that will make it possible to understand the specific situation of the practice. For example, a telephone analysis can show all of the following:

- The peak hours for volume of calls
- How quickly calls are answered
- How long patients wait on the phone
- Where the calls end up—that is, who deals with the call (nurse, referral clerk, or other person)
- The percentage of blocked calls (ie, patients are unable to get through, due to all lines being busy)

How this information is obtained depends on the specifics of the phone system. Some systems will keep track of this information automatically and provide monthly (or even weekly) data; some local phone companies provide much of this information on a periodic basis; and, in many offices, particularly smaller ones that have basic phone systems, the information can be obtained manually.

Using this data, it is possible to make basic decisions such as how many lines to have (and how many should be incoming and outgoing), what the appropriate phone staffing should be during various times of the week, and what other solutions might help to ensure prompt phone access. Moreover, the data should be collected regularly to assess the impact of interventions to improve the situation [9]. For example, it might be discovered that a disproportionate number of phone calls are due to prescription refills. This can be addressed in a variety of ways, including nontelephone interventions such as encouraging physicians to prescribe chronic medications for longer periods of time (eg, 1 year of hypertension medications rather than 6 months for controlled patients, thus cutting those calls in half) and developing a place on the Web site for patients to request refills (to incorporate this method into the practice, patients will need to be encouraged to use the site and someone at the office will need to check the site at least once a day for these requests). An example of a telephone-based intervention is the use of an automated voice attendant that allows patients to push a number and be routed directly to a voice mailbox where they can leave their request and thus do not have to wait; a staff member then checks the voice mailbox multiple times daily.

Another option that a site may wish to consider to improve telephone access is to have a call center, especially if they want to have a live person answer the phone. The call center usually is located away from the front desk to provide privacy and eliminate the distraction of patients coming and going [9]. The benefit of a call center is that it provides a live human to answer every call and address the needs of the patient directly (such as making an appointment or routing the call to the appropriate place). In addition, because individuals who run the call center are highly focused and can be taught specific phone-related customer service methods, they can become quite skilled at managing the phones, with a resultant increase in patient satisfaction. Call centers usually are found in larger offices, but smaller practices can hire one person who answers the phone and has no other responsibilities to distract them.

Other interventions for improving telephone access also are available. Many of these fall under the category of reducing unnecessary phone calls. For example, let's look at phone calls for nursing advice. In the past, the patient would request to speak with the nurse. The clerk would take the message, go pull the chart, put the message on the chart, and then place the chart and the message in the nurse's box. The nurse would get the chart and call the patient back when she had time. In the meantime, many patients would call back because the nurse was delayed in getting back to them, resulting in additional calls. If the nurse takes the call "live," however—that is, when the patient calls—the number of future phone calls from anxious patients will be reduced. In addition, with the increasing use of computers for patient information, it is no longer necessary to pull a chart, thus freeing up the clerk even more to answer other calls more promptly.

The Internet provides similar options for reducing unnecessary phone. One simple intervention is to have an online referral request page, as well as a prescription refill request page. Some larger medical institutions are beginning to experiment with patient portals. A patient portal is basically a way in which patients are given more direct access to their medical records and their physicians via the Internet. The University of Michigan Medical Center is working on a patient portal that will allow patients to directly e-mail their physicians with any questions, view their laboratory results, and eventually even make appointments. Clearly, patient portals have the potential to reduce significantly the number of phone calls for those who can afford them; however, a variety of problems still need to be worked out, such as being compliant with the Health Insurance Portability and Accountability Act (HIPAA). In the future, more extensive use of the Web undoubtedly will exist.

With regard to telephones, it is important to provide two words of caution: First, setting the vision and then working with the staff to meet the vision is critical. This allows staff to later work through the inevitable glitches of a new system. Second, technology is not a panacea, and in fact can result in new problems [14], which will need to be worked through, and may require adjusting the process or plan. Changing the original plan—based on careful evaluation of the data—is fine, as long as it results in the desired outcome.

SCHEDULING AND MAKING APPOINTMENTS

Although making appointments is part of the initial contact with the office, scheduling is so critical, complex, and, sometimes, difficult to fix [1], that we have made it a separate section. How patients are scheduled traditionally has been the purview of the physician. It is common for each physician in a practice to have different ways in which they want their patients scheduled. This situation creates much confusion for the clerical staff in booking patients and actually can limit access. Larger practices sometimes use dedicated appointment clerks to streamline the process [1]; however, there still are numerous issues, as enumerated below. Even in solo practices, scheduling mechanics can have an enormous impact on access.

The classic format for scheduling was to put patients down for a slot sometime in the future. Eventually, the appointment times filled up, leaving no time for sick patients who called and wanted to be seen the same day. One of the first amendments to this schedule was the wave system, and subsequently, the modified wave (Table 1). The concept behind these systems was that patients often do not show up right on time. Thus, waiting for a patient who is 10 minutes late for a 15-minute appointment can put a physician behind for the rest of the day. The wave approach schedules two 15-minute patients every half hour. Whichever one comes first is seen first. The modified wave has a long and a short at the top of the hour, another short one at 15 minutes after the hour, and then a "long" appointment at half past the hour. Forty-five minutes past the hour is left open for catch-up and overbooks.

TABLE 1.
Examples of Different Schedules[a]

	Wave Schedule	Modified Wave	Carve-Outs[b]	Open Access
9:00	Long visit[c] Short visit[d]	Long visit Short visit	Scheduled	Fill in about 30% of the schedule and the rest of the time is filled in using 1 min for short visits and 30 min for long ones. It does not matter which time slots are filled in ahead of time and which are left open for same-day appointments.
9:15	(Left empty)	Short visit	Scheduled	
9:30	Long visit Short visit	Short or long visit	Scheduled	
9:45	(Left empty)	(Left empty)	Scheduled	
10:00	Long visit Short visit	Long visit Short visit	Scheduled	
10:15	(Left empty)	Short visit	Scheduled	
10:30	Long visit Short visit	Short or long visit	Scheduled	
10:45	(Left empty)	(Left empty)	Scheduled	
11:00	Long visit Short visit	Long visit Short visit	Acute same day Visits only	
11:15	(Left empty)	Short visit	Acute same day Visits only	
11:30	Long visit	Short or long visit	Acute same day visit only	
	Short visit	Short visit	Visits only	
11:45	(Left empty)	(Left empty)	Acute same day Visit only	

[a] Assuming 15-minute schedule blocks for short visits and 30 minutes for long visits.
[b] This is an example of a carve-out for urgent care visits. The same can be done for other types of visits, as needed by the practice.
[c] A long visit is a more complex visit, such as a patient coming in for an HME, abdominal pain, or fatigue.
[d] A short visit is a simpler visit, such as a patient coming in for an ear infection, urinary infection, or rash.

These systems helped some sites, but there still were significant access issues for a variety of situations, in particular, the need to accommodate urgent, same-day visits. Some offices hired nurses to perform phone triage to reduce the number of patients actually seen in the office as well as to help determine how long the visit needed to be, and so forth [15]; this is still a widely used resource [13]. The next generation of scheduling to address the problem of access for same-day visits was to develop carve-out time periods (see Table 1) for urgent care; that is, save a block of appointment times for patients who needed to be seen quickly [8]. Although carve-out periods are an improvement over the traditional method, schedules eventually still get filled and overflow; moreover, this process falsely assumes that the triage system for identifying who is truly urgent works 100% of the time and it does not deal with access for routine care [8], which results in patients being seen by other physicians and at other sites (eg, Emergency Rooms). Moreover, the resulting schedules also can become very complex because there often are other dedicated slots for HMEs, procedures, and other specific types of visits.

The third-generation effort to improve scheduling that was developed is now known as the open-access model, and is defined below (see Table 1). In short, it focuses on seeing patients the day they call and maximizes continuity of care. Places that have implemented open-access scheduling have noted significantly improved patient access, physician satisfaction, and revenue; and, in the end, increased patient satisfaction [7,16].

A specific example of implementing an open-access schedule can be provided by the situation at the University of Michigan health centers (which range in size from small three FTE practices to large multispecialty practices). Until recently, physicians at each site had their own template. This included how long they wanted to see different types of patients, how many HMEs they would see each day, what times they saw HMEs, and so forth. Even within the same office and specialty, there were enormous differences among physicians, which resulted in several outcomes. First, the clerical staff had to remember each physician's desires, or, even after it was programmed into the computer, which physicians would allow exceptions for which situations. In addition, the hundreds of templates programmed into the computer slowed the scheduling system down, and because many physicians would see HMEs only in certain time slots, and urgent care only in other slots, enormous access problems were created. People who wanted HMEs could not get in for long periods of time because all the HME slots were taken and those who wanted to be seen the same day often were sent to the Emergency Room because of lack of appointment times. Moreover, there was a significant no-show rate for many appointments, because patients forgot about their appointment (or neglected to cancel when they got a reminder a day or two before because they had forgotten and scheduled something else during that time). This resulted in reduced access and reduced revenue.

The first step to address the situation was to get all the health centers and departments to agree on the use of common nomenclature. This concept involves all physicians in any particular specialty agreeing on the various appointment types and lengths. Part of this process also focuses on reducing the total number of appointment types. This process is not easy, but it works [10]. For example, the common nomenclature standards that we came up with for primary care at the University of Michigan (Table 2), in effect, reduced the number of scheduling categories from hundreds to approximately 30. This, in turn, resulted in three benefits. First, it greatly simplifies the scheduling process and thus saves time for the clerical staff. If a physician wants more time for a particular patient, they simply request more blocks of an existing category (eg, if a physician wants to schedule a 30-minute appointment, then the scheduler would book two 15-minute visit blocks) rather than have a separate category. Second, the computer system works faster, thus further shortening the time needed to make the appointment. Finally, it has made it easier for the fill-in staff to cover for sick and vacation time, because the scheduling across all sites is the same.

TABLE 2.
University of Michigan Hospital and Health Centers Common Nomenclature Standards for Family Medicine

Standard Appointment Type	Appointment Length	Optional Appointment Type	Appointment Length
NP	30 min	Consult-15	15 min
NP-Urgent	15 min	Consult-30	30 min
NP-HME	30 min	Consult-45	45 min
NP-WCE	30 min	NP-HME-45	45 min
RV	15 min	NP-HME-60	60 min
RV-Urgent	15 min	PROC-30	30 min
RV-HME	30 min	PROC-45	45 min
RV-WCE	30 min	PROC-60	60 min
		PROC-COLP	45 min
		PROC-SIG	45 min
		PROC-VASC	60 min
		RV-30	30 min
		RV-45	45 min
		RV-HME-45	45 min
		RV-HME-60	60 min
		OB-INIT	Site specific
		OB-INIT-RN	Site specific
		RV-OB	15 min
		SPCMPHY	31 min

The next step we instituted was to gradually convert the practices to an open-template schedule. This means that the physician does not specify specific times for various activities. Returning to our HME example above, this would mean that the clerk could put an HME in any time during the day rather than only in certain slots. To prevent burnout, some schedulers place a limit on the total number of HMEs in a day per physician, but not on what times they are scheduled. Similarly, there are no urgent care or other specified slots. The clerk has the ability to put a patient down whenever a spot is available. This increases access in several ways. One, it reduces the amount of time it takes a clerk to schedule a patient because he does not have to search for the next available specified slot for the specific care that the patient is requesting (eg, HME). Two, the clerk does not have to get approval to book a patient with one problem in a spot reserved for another problem. It also has created significant patient satisfaction because they can be seen quickly.

The third, and most visionary alteration in scheduling, the idea of open access, is just beginning to be instituted in some practices at the University of Michigan. The basic concept of open access is that patients are seen the day that they call and are seen by their physician [7]. Once a practice is on an open-access schedule, most patients do not have to book appointments ahead of time. Studies have shown that, contrary to what one might think, this approach does not cause significant overload of physician practices. On the contrary, based on past experience it is possible to predict how many patients will call on any given day and, by leaving the appropriate number of open slots in the schedule on those days, a scheduler can make accommodations for these patients. Waiting lists or backlog for patients to schedule appointments usually are stable and in equilibrium, which suggests that if the backlog was eliminated, the physicians in the practice could then see all their patients promptly. This is not always the case, however (see below), and thus analysis is required to predict accurately the volume of patients and staffing needed [4]. Practices that have performed analyses, determined that they could initiate an open-access schedule, and then converted to such a system have found that physicians actually are more productive, due to a minimal number of no-shows (ie, patients who call that day most likely will come in) [7]; and have higher patient satisfaction [5,6].

How does a practice transition to an open-access schedule? There are several articles that list the process [8,12], but basically it involves a commitment by the physicians to making the change and analyzing demand and the capacity of the practice. Once this occurs, the actual process involves first reducing the backlog of appointments (ie, work extra to see all those patients who need to be seen until the schedules open up). In addition, a change to using fewer appointment types, developing contingency plans, and reducing demand for unnecessary visits also should be implemented. Examples of reducing demand for unnecessary visits include providing preventive care (eg, Papanicolaou's tests, blood pressure checks, and so forth) when patients are being seen for other reasons and scheduling return visits at longer intervals when appropriate [8]. One key action, as mentioned earlier, is predicting the volume of patients and staff for a particular day and month. This step requires time; is abetted by having electronic scheduling [4], which can calculate average volumes from previous months and years much more easily; and often is done using pre-existing protocols. However, each practice is different (eg, those in southern climates will have less variability than do those in northern climates), and, even after accounting for these differences, only an estimate can be obtained. Because there will be some variation from the predictions initially, physicians will need to be malleable [4]. Another key assumption here is that there is a relatively stable and realistic panel size. For most practices, open access does not result in excessive numbers of new patients overwhelming the practice. However, in a few situations, this can happen. Thus, a rapidly growing practice that already is full, in a community that is growing rapidly, will not be able to implement an open-access schedule unless they are closed to new patients, expand their hours, or add new physicians. Similarly, a practice with too large a panel size will not be able to accommodate the demand. Thus, understanding the demand for services is critical before deciding to transition to an open-access model [9,17]. At one of the University of Michigan sites, for example, the physicians were very interested in changing to an open-access model. However, an analysis of the practice and market showed that even if the physicians worked extra to reduce their backlog, the panel sizes and demand was such that it would take an additional two physicians before a steady state was reached. Otherwise, converting to an open-access schedule would result in more demand than slots available.

Finally, some pioneering practices have piloted the concept of group visits—sometimes called shared medical visits. In this scenario, a group of patients are seen together at one time and all the patients learn from each other. For example, a physician could have 10 diabetic patients come for a group visit. Each patient could have their hemoglobin A1C drawn before the visit and the results could be available for the physician at the group visit. The group visit itself would last an hour, with the physician talking about the disease for 10 minutes, then a dietician reviewing diet for 10 minutes, followed by 30 minutes of group discussion. The last 10 minutes are reserved for brief individual examinations in private rooms as necessary. Group visits have been quite successful, with high patient satisfaction (patients not only get to spend an hour with the doctor, but also learn from others in the group). They also increase access, because 10 patients are seen in 1 hour rather than in 2.5 to 3 hours. Before implementing group visits, it may be helpful to check out one of the many articles on the subject or the Institute for Health Care Improvement Web site [18]. Keep in mind that to bill for all of these patients, you still need to meet the documentation guidelines. At the University of Michigan, we started group visits in selected practices in the year 2003.

PEOPLE ISSUES

Adding a Web site, making changes to improve the management of phone calls, and changing to an open-access schedule should make significant inroads into reducing access problems. Nevertheless, these interventions, as well as those discussed later in this article, are dependent on people. Staffing a medical office is not a simple affair. This section focuses on staffing decisions specifically from the perspective of maximizing access, keeping in mind that numerous parameters are involved, and staffing decisions affect other areas (eg, margin and space allocation).

To begin with, there needs to be adequate numbers of staff, including enough people answering the phones to meet the types and volume of calls for the particular practice. Conducting an analysis of phone call variation throughout the day should allow the management team to better decide how to deploy telephone staffing throughout the office hours. In addition, staffing may vary; for example, Monday mornings often are one of the busiest times of the week, whereas Tuesday afternoons may be relatively slow. Therefore, an office may have an extra person answering the phones on Monday mornings but on Tuesday afternoons have her doing other things or working part time.

Remember, the appropriate staffing for maximizing access should be viewed in a broader context—that is, not just in the context of who actually is answering the phone. For example, some offices have a specific nurse triage line, whereas others do not. The former might be able to justify a higher percentage of nurses on their staff. Similar analysis should be undertaken with the other aspects of the practice, including dedicating a person whose job is to periodically check patient voicemail boxes and Web site prescription or other refill sites, and call patients for follow-up [19].

Likewise, having enough personnel to move patients through the office is critical. Adequate front desk staff who check patients in and verify information as necessary, as well as medical assistant (MA) support is key. There are multiple benchmarks for these positions, depending on the specialty and size of the office. One point needs to be stressed. The more jobs that can be delegated to nonphysician persons, the more time the physicians can spend seeing patients, and thus the more patients who theoretically can be seen. Most efficient offices have at least one MA for each physician; some extremely busy physicians even use two. Specific protocols that ensure that the MAs do as much as they can before the patient sees the physician help to free up valuable physician time to see patients; for example, an MA can perform a visual acuity test for any patient with an eye complaint or obtain a urinalysis for any patient with abdominal discomfort. Depending on the specific needs of the practice, MAs also can do many other tasks. Although many offices commonly have MAs perform such duties as drawing blood, performing bench laboratories, calling in prescriptions, writing (or, in computer-savvy offices, printing) refill prescriptions for physician signature, and getting consultants on the phone, it is possible to have them do even more. One of the University of Michigan sites decided to focus on smoking cessation. They had their MAs document whether each patient smoked, and if the patient did smoke, obtain some baseline information to assess the patient's readiness to quit that was available for the physician to review when he or she entered the room.

Higher-level staff also can be used to free up physician time to see more patients. Licensed practical nurses (LPNs) and registered nurses (RNs) often do telephone triage, using specific protocols developed that determine whether sore throats, urinary tract infections, and similar conditions can be treated over the phone rather than having the patients come in for an office visit—a more common scenario in offices that are in heavily managed care environments. However, having LPNs and RNs triage patients can benefit noncapitated situations as well by freeing physicians to see sicker patients. The above-mentioned smoking cessation project had the RNs providing most of the counseling to patients who were ready to quit, after the patients received encouragement from their physician during a brief visit; this freed up the physician to then see other patients.

When discussing appropriate staffing, two other options need to be considered to increase access in extremely busy practices. The first is hiring physician extenders—mainly nurse practitioners (including midwives) and physician assistants. These persons are less expensive than bringing another physician on board, and can see the low-complexity problems such as upper respiratory infections and HMEs (thus allowing physicians to care for more complex patients in a day and increasing the total capacity of the practice). Their presence adds a level of complexity to the entire practice, however, that needs to be considered when making the decision of whether to add them. Several issues need to be discussed: (1) some insurance companies will not pay for care rendered by these providers; (2) depending on the skill of the physician extender in working independently, the physicians may find themselves doing so much oversight that it actually decreases the efficiency of the practice; (3) the rest of the staff has to be educated on what types of patients are appropriate for these providers; (4) in academic settings, these providers might not be appropriate because of the emphasis on teaching students and residents. The second option is to add another physician. Although this option will increase physician access, it likewise has obvious specific issues that need to be evaluated making such a decision.

Finally, adequate training of staff is imperative to ensure that all interventions implemented result in improved efficiency and access. Examples, such as the need for training MAs in tasks that help to increase physician time for patient care, were discussed above. Staff behaviors and attitudes also are important. For instance, if the staff do not arrive in time to be ready for the start of patient care, then patients are not brought back as scheduled, phones are not answered promptly, and the physicians are unable to see as many patients as they otherwise would. Similarly, stocking the rooms, ordering supplies, and other activities need to be performed in such a way as to not slow the physician down. Whether the staff is trained and expectations are set via in-services, visiting model offices to observe, or attending courses needs to be decided by each office.

PHYSICIAN BEHAVIORS

Any attempt to increase access will fail if the physicians are not committed to the process. The case for increasing access needs to be made by the senior physician, medical director of the office, department chair, hospital medical director, or whoever is in charge. In addition to supporting the activities enumerated in this article, physicians often need to change some of their behaviors.

One important factor is that the physician, like the staff, needs to start on time. Starting late is a common reason for physicians falling behind and thus being unable to see add-on or overbooked patients. One common cause for coming to the office late is performing rounds at the hospital. Physicians should assess honestly the time commitment it takes to make their rounds and start hospital rounds early enough so that they can get to the office on time. The demands of the hospital can impact physician access in other ways as well. Calls from nurses with regard to patients often need to be answered during office hours, thus pulling physicians from the examination room allowing for less time to see patients. At times, physicians even may have to go over to the hospital to care for sick patients. Depending on their interest in hospital medicine, the location of their practice, and whether they specialize in obstetrics, some physicians increase their office access to patients by using hospitalists. Hospitalists are physicians who care for patients only in the hospital. Once the patient is discharged, the patient returns to the primary physician. Studies suggest that hospitalists actually decrease length of stay, increase patient satisfaction, and lower overall costs. Primary care physicians who use hospitalists experience increased satisfaction; increased access to patients in their office; and, in some cases, increased revenue.

Another physician-specific factor is the length of visits. The significant variation in this factor appears to be due, in large part, to practice style [20]. With the steadily decreasing payment for medical services and the increasing demand for physician productivity by many institutions, there may be less tolerance of this variability. Learning to see patients more efficiently is a difficult task; how this is accomplished needs to be determined; that is, whether financial incentives, dictates, or some other method is used.

Frequency of return visits, on the other hand, may be a more easily addressable issue. There is significant variation among physicians on this factor, including physicians who are in the same office and whose patients have similar demographics. Lengthening the amount of time for return visits may be an appropriate strategy for some—for example, seeing hypertensive patients who are controlled every 6 to 12 months, rather than every 3 to 4 months. A change in the return visit frequency can yield major improvements in access to appointment slots. In one of the University of Michigan offices that was experiencing dramatic access problems with waits of up to 6 months for some physicians, the medical director consciously began to extend the time period for return visits of stable patients. The time to the third available appointment with him (ie, after filling the first two requests for an appointment, how long it will take the third caller to get an appointment with the doctor) improved within 1 month from 45 to 8 days.

Finally, continuity of care can increase efficiency of care by physicians [21]. Up to 50% of visits to new physicians could be eliminated if patients saw their usual physician [22]. Thus, many offices have pushed for continuity because they believe it increases access in the belief that physicians can see more patients in a defined time period [9]. Continuity is difficult to achieve in some offices in which the physicians have multiple other demands, such as in academic practices. However, when possible, aligning schedules such that physicians are available most days of the week to see their own patients should promote access.

TIME USE

We have already discussed the need for staff and physicians to begin the day on time. This naturally also would apply to beginning any shift after a lunch break. Family physician offices can consider other means of time use to increase access as well—for example, extending the hours of operation. Over the past 50 years, a gradual shift in office hours has occurred. The once-traditional 3-hour (or even shorter) shifts from 9 AM to 12 PM and from 1 PM to 4 PM or 2 PM to 5 PM is not present in most offices now. Instead, the majority of today's offices are open at least 7 hours a day for patient care. If not, then this is an opportunity to increase access.

In addition, so-called extended hours exist in a fair number of places, especially in competitive environments or in locales where a high percentage of both parents work. Extended hours are classically either earlier in the morning (eg, at the University of Michigan we have some sites that start at 7 AM) or later in the day (typically to 6, 7, or 8 PM). It is clear that these hours are popular with patients; the major limitation is convincing physicians to work these hours and then finding employees to staff them.

There are at least two other ways to "extend" office hours without actually incurring the practice expense of beginning earlier or ending later. One is to have appointment slots through the lunch hour (in some clinics, lunch break is even 90 minutes). Depending on the type of patient seen, a significant number of slots can be opened each day by doing so. For example, if three patients were seen during the lunch hour, 5 days a week, that would result in more than 60 patients a month who were accommodated that otherwise would not have been—an increase of 10% or more in accessible time slots.

There are, of course, potential liabilities to having lunch hour appointments that need to be addressed. For one, prevailing laws may require that staff have at least a 15-minute break every 4 hours and an hour break every 6 hours. Moreover, physicians traditionally use this time to dictate, make phone calls, and catch up on their work. Thus, it is necessary to develop creative scheduling of staff and physicians to create this change. Some offices use staggered shifts, such as having one physician work from 8 AM to 12 PM, the next from 10 AM to 2 PM, and so forth. One family practice office that already had evening hours but needed to increase access to patients addressed this problem by having the physicians work 6.5-hour shifts (with a half-hour break in the middle). The practice had nine rooms, yet was able to have four physicians work each day. The shifts were 8 AM to 2:30 PM, 10 AM to 4:30 PM, 11:30 AM to 6 PM, and 1:30 PM to 8 PM. Patients were happy with the increased access, the physicians were happy because they got to spend more time at home, and the practice was able to leverage the fixed expenses to increase significantly the margin for the practice. This example is provided not as a suggestion of an optimal way to schedule patients, but rather to demonstrate that there are alternative ways to maximize the hours.

A second way of extending office hours without incurring an expense to the practice is for a physician to make house calls. These visits are fully billable, pleasing to the patient, and leave an appointment slot open for someone else. In addition, house calls—by giving the physician a better idea of the patient's living situation—often can lead to better care that, down the road, reduces the frequency of visits needed by that patient, thus, further improving access for the practice. Obviously, there are significant negative aspects with house calls that will prevent many physicians from making them—the major one being the time involved, with the concomitant low efficiency.

SPACE

The amount of space and layout of an office can impact access. Some offices, for example, have specialized rooms for procedures or pediatric or gynecologic patients. Such rooms can reduce the efficiency of the office. For example, there may be more than one patient at a time who needs the gynecologic room. In such a situation, the second patient will tie up one of the other examination rooms while waiting for the first patient to be finished (or wait in the reception room and slow the physician down) so that he or she can be moved to the special gynecologic room. It helps to be able to see all types of patients in every room as much as possible. Most procedures can be performed in a regular examination room, including vasectomies.

Time control or operations management experts suggest that patient rooms should not be too large (minimizing extra walking for the physician and patients) and the layout of the rooms should be identical (so that the physician does not have to think about the location of items). This might seem like a small issue, and, on an individual basis, it may be. However, if it saves 30 seconds a patient, multiplied by 20 to 30 patients, it might allow for one additional patient to be seen each day by the physician.

Specific discussion about clinic layout is beyond the scope of this article. In general, where possible, the layout should be configured to minimize the amount of walking for the physicians and staff. Thus, for example, the laboratory (or wherever the microscope is kept) should be centrally located, viewboxes should be easily available, examination rooms should be grouped, and workstations should be contiguous to the examination rooms. Depending on the needs and location of the practice, building additional space always is a potential intervention, although usually a last resort, due to the significant cost involved, both in terms of construction and inconvenience during the remodeling.

MISCELLANEOUS

There are several other factors affecting access that do not fit into the above categories, but should be mentioned. One is the prevailing regulatory environment. The recent implementation of the HIPAA is a typical example. Although not directly related to access, it does place requirements for patient confidentiality that medical offices must follow. Depending on how an office implements these requirements could add extra work for staff, and slow down the process of getting patients ready for the physician.

A second factor is the difficulty that many practices have with obtaining specialty care for their patients. This can result in physicians having to spend time on the phone with the specialist in an attempt to get their patient seen. Improving this process frees physicians to see other patients [9]. Possible ways to help reduce this barrier include developing good relationships with specialists and using alternative methods of communication such as e-mails.

A third factor, for those who work as part of larger institutions, is the ongoing and seemingly ever-increasing cost-reduction campaigns. Physicians need to guard against penny-wise, pound-foolish reductions, such as trying to reduce the MA to physician ratio.

The aging of the baby-boomers is yet another factor that will impact access. As people age, they develop more medical problems, which leads to increased demand for physician contact. Although physicians cannot control the aging of America, awareness of the change might lead to changes in practice that help to maintain access. For example, working with local senior citizen centers to provide on-site blood pressure monitoring, glucose screening, or other high-frequency measurements might lessen the demand for this service in the office. A nonphysician often can perform these procedures. Minimizing rework [5,6] or dead time in the office also can help to improve access [15,23]; unfortunately, a full discussion of this factor is beyond the scope of this article. Lastly, some practices have found that increasing education of their patients has resulted in reduced demand for services [13].

IMPLEMENTATION AND SUMMARY

It is clear that a multitude of areas impact access, some more than others, depending on the practice. Each office or clinic should evaluate their specific situation and decide which interventions would make the biggest impact and be acceptable to the physicians and staff. This article summarizes various interventions that can be implemented with ease. Many of these interventions are based on the size of the practice (Table 3). In general, what works for a large clinic might not work for a solo practice, and vice versa. For example, a solo practice probably will not be able to afford an RN, whereas larger practices are more likely to have the available funds. The data listed in Table 3, however, are only approximations. Each office is unique. This fact is highlighted by the hospitalist option. In concept, a solo-practice physician easily could use a hospitalist in their local hospital, in the process freeing up time to spend in the office. In a rural environment, however, where the physician is the only one in town (as opposed to a solo doctor in a large city), a hospitalist is not an option.

Donald Berwick, MD, the lead physician at the Institute for Health Care Improvement, has pushed for the implementation of a Continuous Quality Improvement (CQI) program [18]. He advocates the well-described Plan-Do-Study-Act (PDSA or PDCA where C stands for check) approach to quality improvement, regardless of the location or type of practice [24]. Basically, he argues that by doing small-scale "experimentations," physicians can make significant changes in an organized and effective manner. In the case of improving access, such an approach would certainly work. A practice, regardless of type, location, or size, could identify a plan, implement it, and then modify it depending on the outcomes. This CQI process of monitoring the results of interventions and making changes as

TABLE 3.
Ease of Implementing Various Access Interventions Based on Size of the Practice Alone

	Telephone Call Analysis	Call Center	Reducing Phone Calls	Open Access	Open Template	Common Nomenclature	Group Visits	Staffing Analysis	RNs	Physician Extenders	Hospitalists Usage	Return Visit Reduction	Continuity of Care	Alternative Hours	Space Changes
Private practice															
1-3 physicians	3	3	2	3	2	1	1	1	3	1	1	1	3	2	3
4-7 physicians	1	2	1	3	2	2	1	1	2	1	1	2	3	1	3
8 or more physicians	1	1	1	3	2	3	1	1	1	1	1	3	2	1	3
Academic/institutional practice	1	1	1	3	2	3	1	1	1	2	1	3	1	2	3

1 = easiest; 3 = hardest.

indicated has proved to be beneficial in multiple situations, including health care environments [9,25].

The Appendix at the end of this article is a check-off sheet that lists the interventions that have been discussed. Physicians can use the Appendix, along with Table 3, to decide which interventions might be applicable to their situation. Further information about the various topics discussed above is available via the references listed at the end of this article. Finally, additional information on any item can likewise be obtained from the American Academy of Family Physicians (Leawood, Kansas), the Institute for Health Care Improvement (Boston, Massachusetts), and the Medical Group Management Association (Englewood, Colorado).

Key Points

- This article discusses the issue of improving patient access to the services of family physicians.
- Various factors that impede this access are reviewed, and potential methods to address each of these factors are discussed, taking into account the fact that every practice is unique.
- A check-off form and summary are included for the reader's benefit.

References

[1] Gallagher M, Pearson P, Drinkwater C. Managing patient demand: a qualitative study of appointment making in general practice. 2001;51:280–5.
[2] Schon C. Improving ambulatory care access and service delivery. ACMPE Paper; June: 1999.
[3] Hurst NP, Lambert CM, Forbes J, Lochhead A, Major K, Lock P. Does waiting matter? A randomized controlled trial of new non-urgent rheumatology outpatient referrals. Rheumatology 2000;39:369–76.
[4] Forjuoh SN, Averitt WM, Cauthen DB, Couchman GR, Symm B, Mitchell M. Open-access appointment scheduling in family practice: comparison of a demand prediction grid with actual appointments. J Am Board Fam Pract 2001;14:259–65.
[5] Kilo CM, Endsley S. As good as it could get: remaking the medical practice. Fam Pract Manage 2000;7:48–52.
[6] Kilo CM, Delio SA, Littell F. Office efficiency: managing a high volume practice. Forum 2000;February:31–2.
[7] Boelke C, Boushon B, Isensee S. Achieving open access: the road to improved service and satisfaction. MGMA Journal 2000;47:58–62, 64–6, 68.
[8] Murray M. Patient care: access. BMJ 2000;320:1594–6.
[9] Anctil B, Winters M. Linking customer judgments with process measures to improve access to ambulatory care. Jt Comm J Qual Improv 1996;22:345–57.
[10] Hull B. Service standards hallmark for practice marketing. Medical Group Management Update 1995;34(11):10.
[11] Zablocki E. A change in practice; physicians adopt new methods to eliminate patients' long wait for appointments. Healthplan 2000;November–December:52–4.
[12] Murray M, Tantau C. Same-day appointments: exploding the access paradigm. Fam Pract Manage 2000;7:45–50.
[13] Goldberg SE. Demand management: implementing your own program. Fam Pract Manage 1998;5:49–62.

[14] Mashburn J. Telephone access and telephone system evaluation, selection and implementation of new systems. MGMA Archive, ACMPE Paper, February 2001.

[15] Andrews S, Croes D. For patients and providers, it's all about access. MGMA Journal 1999;46(3):36–40.

[16] Murray M, Tantau C. Redefining excellence in open access to primary care. Manage Care Quarterly 1999;7:45–55.

[17] Reeves K, Anctil E. Improving outpatient appointment access—lessons learned. Ambulatory. Outreach 1997;Winter:10–2.

[18] Institute for Healthcare Improvement website. IDCOP themes. Available at: http/www.ihi.org/idealized/idcop/access.asp. Accessed September 12, 2003.

[19] Bodenheimer T, Lo B, Casalino L. Primary care physicians should be coordinators, not gatekeepers. JAMA 1999;281:2045–9.

[20] Schwartz LM, Woloshin S, Wasson JH, Renfrew RA, Welch HG. Setting the revisit interval in primary care. J Gen Intern Med 1999;14:230–5.

[21] Raddish M, Horn SD, Sharkey PD. Continuity of care: is it cost effective? American Journal of Managed Care 1999;5:727–34.

[22] Weymier R. New trends in patient access. MGMA Journal. APA Matrix 2001;16(1).

[23] Kilo C, Moore LG. Improving access and efficiency in the clinical office. Call 4: key changes for improving office efficiency. IHI 2002;Feb 27.

[24] Berwick DM. Developing and testing changes in delivery of care. Ann Intern Med 1998;128:651–6.

[25] Zazove P, Klinkman M. Developing a CQI program in a family medicine department. Journal of Quarterly Improvement 1998;24(8):391–401.

Address reprint requests to

Department of Family Medicine
University of Michigan Hospital
Ambulatory Care Services
7300 Dexter Ann Arbor Road
Dexter, MI 48130

e-mail: pzaz@umich.edu

APPENDIX

Improving Access Checklist

                                                                                          Yes   No

1. Telephones
    Can a call analysis be done on our phone system?   — —
    If not, will the phone company provide this?   — —
    If not, is there someone in the office who can do manually?   — —
    Number of phone lines adequate?   — —
    Do we want alternative ways for patients to give requests?   — —
    Voice mailbox?   — —
    Web site?   — —
    Should we consider a call center, or dedicated person to answer calls?   — —
    Do our nurses and referral person take calls live?   — —
    If not, should they?   — —

2. Scheduling
  Do we have standardized nomenclature? — —
   If not, should we? — —
  Are the physician schedules designed to maximize — —
   access?
   If not, should they be changed? — —
   If yes, how? — —
    Wave? — —
    Modified wave? — —
    Open template? — —
    Open access? — —
  Would group visits be applicable to our practice? — —
   If so, what topics? — —
3. Staffing
  Are we appropriately staffed overall compared to — —
   benchmarks?
   Do we have peak times that need special — —
    attention?
  What places do we need someone monitoring for — —
   patient input?
   Web site? — —
   Voice mailbox? — —
   Nurse triage? — —
   Referral coordinator? — —
   Other? — —
  Is the MA: physician ratio optimal for access? — —
  Are there enough clerical staff to move patients — —
   through thus allowing maximal access?
  Are there significant opportunities for using RNs and — —
   LPNs to increase access?
  Would adding a physician extender increase access — —
   significantly?
  Do we need to add another physician? — —
  Are adequate training programs in place to ensure — —
   that staff can do their job sufficiently to allow
   maximal access?
4. Physician Behavior
  Do physicians start on time? — —
   If not, why? — —
  Are hospitalists available at the hospital we use? — —
   If so, do we want to utilize them? — —
  Can the length of visits be shortened? — —
  Are physicians willing to: — —
   Schedule follow-up visits at longer intervals for — —
    stable patients?
   Prescribe chronic medications for longer time — —
    periods?

5. Time Utilization

      Does our practice have extended hours?   — —

      If not, should we?   — —

      If so, are they at the appropriate times?   — —

    Do we currently schedule patients during the lunch   — —
      hour?

      If not, should we?   — —

    Do our physicians make house calls?   — —

      If not, should they and, if so, under what   — —
      circumstances?

6. Space

    Do we have specialized rooms?   — —

      If so, do we wish to continue with this?   — —

    Are all the rooms standardized?   — —

    Is the layout of the practice optimal to minimizing   — —
      physician movement?

      Room allocation?   — —

      Viewboxes?   — —

      Office near rooms being used?   — —

      Microscope available near rooms?   — —

      Other?   — —

    Do we wish to expand our space?   — —

      If so, is space available?   — —

7. Are there other areas which impact on patient access?   — —

      If so, are these fixable?   — —

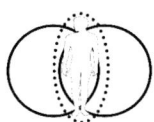

PROFESSIONAL AND PRACTICE MANAGEMENT SKILLS 1522–5720/03 $15.00 + .00

CUMULATIVE INDEX 2003

Volume 5

Note: Page numbers of article titles are in **boldface** type.

YES! Please start my subscription to the **CLINICS** checked below with the ❑ first issue of the calendar year or ❑ current issue. If not completely satisfied with my first issue, I may write "cancel" on the invoice and return it within 30 days at no further obligation.

❑ Bill Me ❑ Check Enclosed ❑ Visa
❑ MasterCard ❑ AmEx

card #____ /____ /____ / exp.____ /____

Signature_____
Make checks payable to **W.B. SAUNDERS**.
Staple this to your purchase order to expedite delivery.

Please Print:

Name_____

Address_____

City_____

State_____ Zip_____

(left margin, vertical) Order your subscription today. Simply complete and detach this card and drop it in the mail to receive the best clinical information in your field.

❑**Anesthesiology**
Quarterly $162
Institutions $230
*Residents $81

❑**Cardiology**
Quarterly $155
Institutions $231
*Residents $76

❑**Chest Medicine**
Quarterly $176
Institutions $241

❑**Chest Surgery**
Quarterly $161
Institutions $219

❑**Child and Adolescent Psychiatric**
Quarterly $161
Institutions $227

❑**Critical Care**
Quarterly $155
Institutions $228
*Residents $78

❑**Dental**
Quarterly $142
Institutions $205

❑**Emergency Medicine**
Quarterly $156
Institutions $228
❑Send CME info

❑**Facial Plastic Surgery**
Quarterly $184
Institutions $263

❑**Foot and Ankle**
Quarterly $147
Institutions $199

❑**Gastroenterology**
Quarterly $176
Institutions $240

❑**Gastrointestinal Endoscopy**
Quarterly $177
Institutions $228

❑**Hand**
Quarterly $188
Institutions $273

❑**Hematology/ Oncology**
Bimonthly $195
Institutions $265

❑**Immunology & Allergy**
Quarterly $156
Institutions $228

❑**Infectious Disease**
Quarterly $155
Institutions $230

❑**Infertility & Reproductive Medicine**
Quarterly $149
Institutions $232
*Residents $75

❑**Clinics in Liver Disease**
Quarterly $155
Institutions $201

❑**Medical**
Bimonthly $130
Institutions $209
*Residents $65
❑Send CME info

❑**MRI**
Quarterly $177
Institutions $249
❑Send CME info

❑**Neuroimaging**
Quarterly $177
Institutions $247
❑Send CME info

❑**Neurologic**
Quarterly $166
Institutions $247

❑**Obstetrics & Gynecology**
Quarterly $162
Institutions $247

❑**Occupational and Environmental Medicine**
Quarterly $110
Institutions $143
*Residents $55

❑**Ophthalmology**
Quarterly $177
Institutions $279

❑**Oral & Maxillo-facial Surgery**
Quarterly $165
Institutions $239

❑**Orthopedic**
Quarterly $172
Institutions $250
*Residents $86

❑**Otolaryngologic**
Bimonthly $188
Institutions $301

❑**Pediatric**
Bimonthly $126
Institutions $209
*Residents $63
❑Send CME info

❑**Perinatology**
Quarterly $142
Institutions $204
❑Send CME info

❑**Plastic Surgery**
Quarterly $224
Institutions $325

❑**Podiatric Medicine & Surgery**
Quarterly $154
Institutions $228

❑**Primary Care**
Quarterly $126
Institutions $191

❑**Psychiatric**
Quarterly $159
Institutions $247

❑**Radiologic**
Bimonthly $205
Institutions $284
*Residents $102
❑Send CME info

❑**Sports Medicine**
Quarterly $167
Institutions $238

❑**Surgical**
Bimonthly $176
Institutions $256
*Residents $88

❑**Urologic**
Quarterly $179
Institutions $263
❑Send CME info

BUSINESS REPLY MAIL

FIRST-CLASS MAIL   PERMIT NO. 7135   ORLANDO FL

POSTAGE WILL BE PAID BY ADDRESSEE

PERIODICALS ORDER FULFILLMENT DEPT
WB SAUNDERS
ELSEVIER SCIENCE
6277 SEA HARBOR DRIVE
ORLANDO FL 32821-9816